Medicine for Sport

Medicine for Sport

by

David F. Apple, Jr., M.D.

Medical Director of the Shepherd Center
for the Treatment of Spinal Injuries
Atlanta, Georgia
Team Physician, Atlanta Hawks

and

John D. Cantwell, M.D.

Director of the Preventive Cardiology Clinic
and Co-director of Cardiac Rehabilitation
Georgia Baptist Hospital
Atlanta, Georgia
Team Physician, Atlanta Braves

YEAR BOOK MEDICAL PUBLISHERS, INC.
CHICAGO · LONDON

Library of Congress Cataloging in Publication Data

Apple, David F
  Medicine for sport.

  Includes index.
  1. Sports medicine. I. Cantwell, John D., joint
author. II. Title. [DNLM: 1. Sport medicine
QT260 A648 m]
RC1210.A66   617'.1027   79-14362
ISBN 0-8151-1422-2

To my family who supported the effort required and were understanding of the time involved.

DAVID F. APPLE, JR., M.D.

To my former coaches:

WILLIAM AND ARTHUR CANTWELL

Who taught me how to angle punts into the coffin corner on the vacant lot next door.

SALLY CANTWELL BASTING

Who taught her baby brother how to fight back when cornered.

JOHN KENNEY

Who combined discipline and a dry wit to guide the Shawano Indians to consecutive state basketball championships.

VIC BUBAS

Who emphasized the importance of a burning desire and led the Duke Blue Devils to the 1960 Atlantic Coast Conference title.

JOHN D. CANTWELL, M.D.

Preface

This book is not a textbook of sports medicine. As physicians who work with amateur and professional athletes, we have attempted to write a simple monograph that will be useful to team physicians, trainers, health educators and to athletes themselves. We highlight some of our experiences in the diagnosis and treatment of common musculoskeletal problems, general medical conditions, cardiovascular diseases and mimics of diseases. We also emphasize selected aspects of exercise physiology and describe some basic aspects of nutrition. Since the doctor who works with athletes is often asked to give advice on physical fitness, we have presented our viewpoint on this timely topic.

Team physicians are often former athletes who retain an interest in sports and who enjoy working with dynamic people. Team doctors should strive to practice high-quality medicine and should avoid catering to the whims of the athlete who requests vitamin B_{12} injections, anabolic steroids or "diet pills." They should not tolerate the inappropriate use by paramedical personnel of antibiotics for colds and sore throats. One cultures the throat of an office patient who complains of soreness to determine whether pathogenic bacteria are present. The same practice should apply to the evaluation and therapy of the athlete who is seen in the locker room.

We are encouraged by the growing enthusiasm for participation in sports by all age groups during the past few years. For example, amateur adult softball players increased from 16 million in 1970 to 26 million in 1976. In 1976, Americans spent $960 million on bicycles. Within the last 4 years tennis equipment sales have escalated from $78 million to $666 million. The enthusiasm for running and jogging can be seen in urban neighborhoods which at dawn are often dotted with jogging men, women and children, most of whom have experienced the joy of being physically fit for the first time in their lives. Physicians themselves have joined the ranks; in fact, 10% of the participants in the 1978 Boston Marathon were physicians. National medical organizations for the jogger, tennis player, skier and others have been formed.

Increased participation will inevitably produce more sports-related medical problems, and specialists in this field are a welcome addition to the medical ranks. We hope this book will assist and encourage those involved in medicine for sports, and we hope that they will enjoy the experience as much as we have.

DAVID F. APPLE, JR., M.D.

JOHN D. CANTWELL, M.D.

Acknowledgments

The musculoskeletal chapters of this volume underwent the valuable scrutiny of Edward C. Loughlin, Jr., M.D., and Joe O'Toole, registered physical therapist and athletic trainer. Patsy Bryan meticulously created the anatomical drawings, and Bob Beveridge reproduced them for publication. Miss Leslie Hudson ably assisted with the syntax. The final review was performed by my former teacher, Gladys Hoffman, and is greatly appreciated.

DAVID F. APPLE, JR., M.D.

I would like to thank Edward W. Watt, Ph.D., David Martin, Ph.D. and Sara Hunt, R.D., Ph.D. for their critical comments.

JOHN D. CANTWELL, M.D.

Contents

1 / Physical Fitness

We are a nation of nonexercisers, for the most part. In 1974, a survey was conducted by the President's Council on Physical Fitness and Sports to determine just how much and what kinds of exercise Americans engage in. The findings were astounding: approximately 45% of adult Americans did not participate in any form of exercise, yet 57% of those sampled thought they were getting more than enough physical exercise. Nearly two thirds of the nonexercisers thought they were as physically fit as they ought to be.

Of the 60 million adults who said they did exercise, the most popular activities were as follows:

Walking	44 million
Bicycling	18 million
Swimming	14 million
Calisthenics	14 million
Jogging	6 million

More than half of the walkers did so almost daily, but few of those who said they participated in other forms of exercise did so with any degree of regularity.

The President's survey listed the various types of group sports that American adults prefer. Bowling (20%) and swimming (18%) were the most favored, followed by golf (9%), softball (8.5%) and tennis (6%).

Who should bear the blame for the rather pitiful state of our nation's physical fitness? While the survey did not provide a

Portions of this chapter were published in *Pulse* (Vol. 1, no. 2, 1977, used with permission of the editor) and were presented at the conference on exercise in the elderly (National Heart, Lung and Blood Institute, Washington, D.C., Oct. 29, 1977).

specific answer to this question, it did indicate that 80% of those questioned had never been advised by their physicians to participate in regular physical activity. Even when the physician did state that a patient should "get a little exercise," the type, frequency, intensity or duration was rarely indicated.

Over the past decade or so, we have come to the conclusion that exercise needs to be prescribed for patients just as one prescribes drugs. A doctor doesn't dump a handful of pills into a patient's lap and tell him or her to "take a few"; on the contrary, he specifies the dose and the frequency. The same should apply to exercise.

OUR VAST EXERCISE POTENTIAL

Before we discuss the benefits of exercise and the exercise prescription, let us briefly consider the phenomenal capacity of the human organism for such activity. It is difficult for the average person to do 100 consecutive sit-ups or 50 push-ups; yet the world records for these activities are around 27,000 and 7,000, respectively. While some individuals complain about having to walk several blocks to the grocery store, Capt. Alan Jones swam the length of the Mississippi River (at 50 miles per day); Ken Crutchlow ran 145 miles from Death Valley to the 14,495-foot peak of Mt. Whitney.

There are some remarkable examples of high fitness levels in old age. Noel Johnson started his fitness program at age 70 and now, 6 years later, holds the record for long-distance events in the 70–75 age group of the AAU Masters Program.

Ernie Williamson (Fig 1–1) aged 73, was a high-school and college track performer but was relatively inactive for nearly 40 years thereafter. Upon his retirement at age 63, he started a walking program, building up to 20 miles per day. He first tried jogging at age 68 and had difficulty going 100 yards. However, over a 10-month period he rapidly enhanced his tolerance to a point where he could slowly jog 10 miles per day. In less than 5 years he has run over 10,000 miles and, at this writing, continues to average 10 miles per day.

One of the authors (JDC) was delighted to discover a softball league, the "Kids and Kubs," in St. Petersburg, Florida, for

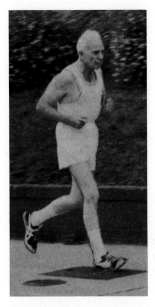

Fig 1–1.—75-year-old Ernie Williamson, who began jogging at age 68 and currently covers 10 miles per day.

those over age 75. One of the players maintained a hefty batting average and was a threat on the base paths as long as his pacemaker was functioning well. Another player, 88-year-old Jim Walche, expressed enthusiasm for the program: "You lay down [*sic*], you die. I believe a lot of us wouldn't be living if we weren't playing ball down here." The oldest player on the team, 97-year-old John Maloney, was asked about his pitching prowess and replied: "I put a little spin on the ball and make the batter hit it into the ground. Nobody makes home runs against me. They say if I could just pitch a little faster, no one would even get a hit off me."[1]

THE BENEFITS OF EXERCISE

Scientists are still not sure that regular exercise prevents heart attacks or that it lengthens life, but two things are quite clear:

1. Regular exercise makes the heart, lungs and vascular system *function better.*
2. Exercise makes one *feel better.*

The improvement in cardiovascular function has been well documented by exercise testing before and after completion of a fitness program. Exercise enhances the body's ability to utilize oxygen, which helps to fuel body functions.

A physically fit person tends to have a lower pulse rate and blood pressure level after a given amount of work than does an untrained person. Stated another way, regular exercise reduces the energy requirements of the heart muscle. This concept can be compared to that of a properly tuned car's getting more miles to a gallon of gasoline.

Psychological tests have confirmed subjective expressions of less depression and anxiety and a better self-image after participation in a physical fitness program.

There are other benefits as well. Over the past 5 years, one of us (JDC) has collected data on 835 persons (730 men, 105 women) without known heart disease who underwent treadmill exercise testing with oxygen uptake analysis and who were given exercise prescriptions. The average age of the men was 40.7 years and of the women, 38.7 years. Two thirds were between the ages of 30 and 49, and 18% were over age 50. Their fitness classes were divided into 7 groups, based on oxygen uptake levels specified by the American Heart Association. The relationship between fitness level and certain parameters, such as aerobic points earned per week, lipid levels, body composition and lung function were examined. When the very low fitness group (144 persons) was compared with the high fitness group (138 persons), the following differences were noted:

| | FITNESS CLASS | |
	VERY LOW	HIGH
Weight (lb)	195.8	166.9°
Body fat (%)	22.1	14.9°
Cholesterol (mg/100 cc)	233.1	220.5
Triglycerides (mg/100 cc)	180.2	100.4°
Blood pressure (rest) (mm Hg)		
Systolic	136.7	129.0°
Diastolic	89.3	81.5°
Blood pressure (exercise) (mm Hg)		
Systolic	186.7	178.7°°
Diastolic	89.5	81.3°

°p < .001 compared to very low group.
°°p < .01 compared to very low group.

In other words, persons in the high fitness group had fewer coronary risk factors than those in the very low fitness group. This does not prove that exercise was the sole reason for the risk factor difference; diet may have played a role.

Kasch and his colleagues[2] found that regular physical exercise in middle age and beyond can counter the tendency for one's maximum oxygen uptake to decline with advancing age. Hence, what was thought by some to be a "normal" phenomenon of the aging process may merely be the "rusting" process of unused organs. Indeed, we studied a 70-year-old jogger and found his maximum oxygen intake to be nearly 55 milliliters oxygen per kilogram of body weight per minute,[3] considerably higher than the reading of 42 ml/kg/min we once observed in a Georgia Tech football halfback who was 50 years younger! Maybe one can stay "young at heart."

THE EXERCISE PRESCRIPTION

In prescribing exercise for an individual middle-aged or older, it is important first to take a thorough medical history and then to perform a physical examination. A resting ECG should be followed by an exercise test, using a stationary bicycle or a treadmill, to see how the heart performs under stress. If there are no signs of heart rhythm disturbances or of insufficient blood supply to heart muscle (which can be indirectly ascertained from the exercise ECG), the patient is given an exercise prescription based on the concept of the "target heart rate," discussed on page 10.

CHARACTERISTICS OF PHYSICAL FITNESS

Physical fitness has 4 components, which can be remembered by the acronym SAFE:

    S = strength
    A = ability (or skill)
    F = flexibility
    E = endurance

In this section, we will discuss only strength, flexibility and endurance, since it is the development of these elements, together with any resulting problems, that is of primary concern in the field of sports medicine.

Strength

Strength is the ability to produce tension in the muscle; power is the rapidity with which this tension can be developed. Muscle strength increases until approximately age 30 and gradually decreases thereafter. This degeneration occurs earlier, and perhaps more rapidly, in those who are inactive. If one becomes inactive after working at strength development, it is estimated that the loss in strength will approximate 10% per week.

There are several ways to develop strength. Four principal methods are outlined below.

Isotonic Exercise

In isotonic exercise, resistance is always constant. An example is weightlifting — the lifting of a fixed weight through a full range of joint motion. Because muscles contract at different degrees of maximum throughout the range of motion, the effect of the resistance will be greatest at the extremes of the motion range. In other words, the tension demand is maximal during only a small portion of the motion range. The major limitation of this exercise form is that the load is limited to what the muscles can move at their weakest point in the motion range.

Isometric Exercise

With isometric exercise, the muscle develops tension against resistance but does not shorten. An example is the exertion of force against an immovable object, such as a wall. The problem with this type of exercise is that strength gains occur only in a small range of joint motion (the point in the motion range where force is applied to the wall or other immovable object).

Isokinetic Exercise

In isokinetic exercise, resistance is variable, unlike isotonic exercise. Consequently, maximum tension and strength develop throughout the full range of joint motion. Using a recently developed machine, it is possible to develop maximum tension at variable speeds.

This type of exercise uses only concentric contractions, with little or no resistance during the eccentric contractions or recovery phase.

Exercise With Nautilus Equipment

Exercise with Nautilus equipment provides resistance against a full range of motion, for the resistance can rotate on a common axis with the involved joints. When force pulls against the muscles at the start of a movement (so-called back pressure or negative work), one can prestretch a muscle to get maximum contraction. This negative-work component is not present in isotonic weightlifting or in isokinetic exercise.

Nautilus exercise does not provide a variable load or resistance through the full range of motion. For instance, the load on a knee in the full squat position should be considerably less than when the knee is fully extended. This is not the case in Nautilus, where the load is constant.

Let us consider, then, the advantages and disadvantages of each form of exercise:

ISOTONIC

Advantages	Disadvantages
1. Relatively inexpensive (compared to Nautilus equipment)	1. Resistance does not vary at different points in the range of motion
2. Smaller pieces of equipment	
3. Time-honored way of increasing strength	

ISOMETRIC

1. Cheap	1. Strength gain only occurs in a limited portion of the range of motion
2. Will improve strength	

ISOKINETIC

1. Resistance varies throughout the full range of motion	1. Costly (may exceed $10,000)

NAUTILUS

| 1. Employs prestretching of muscles | 1. Costly ($2,000 – $3,000) |
| | 2. Load doesn't vary throughout the range of motion |

Pipes et al.[4] compared isokinetic with isotonic strength development in 36 adult men, aged 20 – 38 years. Prior to the 8-week training program, the subjects were randomly assigned to one of four groups:

Group 1 – isotonic exercise

Group 2 – isokinetic, low speed (24 degrees of limb movement per second)

Group 3 – isokinetic, high speed (136 degrees of limb movement per second)

Group 4 – control

The isotonic group trained at 75% of their maximum tolerance. Static strength was measured by cable tensiometry (at 90 degrees and 135 degrees of joint angle for elbow flexion and extension, triceps extension, and the simulated bench press). Dynamic strength was measured by the one-rep maximum isotonic contraction and by isokinetic strength. The strength gain in the study was greater in the isokinetic group than in the control or the isotonic group.

Wilmore[5] put 47 women and 26 men through a 10-week weight training program, measuring changes in strength, body composition and anthropometry. He found that, while overall weight did not show a significant decrease, fat weight decreased 7.5% in men and 9.3% in women. Lean body weight increased 2.4% in the men and 1.9% in the women. There was no significant change in subcutaneous fat thickness in the two body areas that were exercised most, confirming earlier findings by Gwinup[6] that one cannot "spot-reduce."

Wilmore noted little difference in lower-extremity strength between boys and girls when their heights were the same. Women's upper bodies were weaker, since they were used less in strength-developing activities. Strength in both men and women improves similarly with weight training. As other studies showed, Wilmore found that muscle hypertrophy was not a consistent result of strength development — a finding that should be encouraging to women who fear that increased strength means increased muscle bulk.

Clarke[7-9] summarized multiple studies on muscle strength, pointing out the fallacy of "muscle-bound" weight lifters (their joint movement speed is actually increased with training). He also noted that baseball players' throwing speed can be increased by both isometric and isotonic training sessions. Weight training may improve the performance of track runners and the vertical jumping of basketball players. As a rule, most studies showed greater strength and endurance gains through isotonic, rather than isometric, exercise.

Another interesting point made in these studies was that strength imbalance between right and left thigh muscles may contribute to knee injuries. In one study, 79.5% of all knee injuries were to the left knee, which was 7.9% weaker than the noninjured knee. The well players had only a 4.7% difference in strength between the muscles of the right and left thigh.

It seems prudent from preliminary studies to compare the strength of right and left hamstring muscle groups and to assess the ratio of quadriceps strength to hamstring strength in both legs. Lee Burkitt, at San Diego State College, studied 30 trackmen and 36 San Diego Charger football players. In those who subsequently developed hamstring pulls, one hamstring characteristically was more than 10% weaker than the other. Those who had no hamstring pulls had less than 10% differences in hamstring strength and also had normal quadriceps-to-hamstring strength ratios of 60:40.[10]

Flexibility

Paul Uram, flexibility coach of the Pittsburgh Steelers, puts players with quad-hamstring strength ratios higher than 60:40 on resistive flexibility exercises. In his five years of working with professional football players, he has had only one player miss a game because of an injury to his hamstring muscle. Little wonder, then, that the Steelers do stretching exercises prior to games, at halftime, and immediately following games.[10]

Endurance

Wilmore and associates[11] performed fitness tests on 185 professional football players, representing 14 teams. Strength, flexibility, endurance and power were assessed. The authors found that the cardiovascular endurance capacity was "the weakest link in the performance profile of the professional football player."

In order to develop a high level of endurance, one needs to perform exercises that elevate the heart rate to between 70 and 85% of the maximum rate for one's age group. This is known as the target heart rate for exercise. The maximum heart rate decreases with age and, accordingly, so will the target heart rate (Table 1-1).

For example, a 50-year-old man with a maximum heart rate of 170 beats per minute on the treadmill test should exercise at an intensity that will raise the pulse to 119-145 beats per min. Each exercise session should last at least 15-20 minutes and should be done 3 to 5 times per week.

Patients with heart disease should confine vigorous activity to medically supervised exercise classes but may walk and do flexibility exercises on their own. Patients with fixed-rate pacemakers should be encouraged to ,walk up to several miles per day and also to keep limber through routine flexibility exercise. They should not jog, cycle at a fast pace or swim laps in a pool. Those with demand pacemakers, who have a normal underlying impulse conduction for the most part and are not prone to other rhythm disturbances, may be given a target heart rate approximately 60-75% of maximum.

TABLE 1-1.—PREDICTED HEART RATES
(BEATS PER MIN)

AGE	MAXIMUM	85% MAXIMUM		70% MAXIMUM
20	200	170	—	140
30	190	162	—	133
40	180	153	—	126
50	170	145	—	119
60	160	136	—	112
70	150	128	—	105

SPORTS AND FITNESS

The President's Council on Physical Fitness and Sports requested evaluations on 14 popular forms of exercise from 7 experts. Each exercise was judged from the standpoint of heart and lung endurance, muscular endurance, muscular strength, flexibility, balance and general well-being (weight control, muscle definition, digestion, sleep). Each panelist graded the 14 types of exercise on a 0- to 3-point scale. For example, an exercise that was of maximum benefit for muscle endurance would get a total score of 21 (3 points from each of the 7 experts). The overall ratings (total scores of each exercise for each element of physical fitness and general well-being) were then tabulated:[12]

EXERCISE	TOTAL RATING
Jogging	148
Bicycling	142
Swimming	140
Skating	140
Handball/Squash	140
Skiing (Nordic)	139
Basketball	134
Skiing (Alpine)	134
Tennis	128
Calisthenics	126
Walking	102
Golf (cart)	66
Softball	64
Bowling	51

SUMMARY

Persons who are physically fit enjoy subjective benefits of enhanced well-being and objective benefits of improved heart and lung function and lowered coronary risk factors. Proper screening is needed before beginning an exercise program, which should be prescribed by a physician, based upon the exercise stress test and the concept of the target heart rate. Patients with heart disease should confine vigorous activity to a medically supervised exercise program.

Even if evidence is lacking that regular exercise will add years to one's life, most will agree that it adds life to one's years. Dale Groom once wrote, "Most of us, brought up in our sedentary comfortable civilization of today, actually develop and use only a fraction of our potential cardiac reserve."[13]

REFERENCES

1. Quoted in "The National Tattler," June 3, 1973, p. 6.
2. Kasch, F. W.: The effects of exercise on the aging process, Phys. Sportsmed. 4:64, 1976.
3. Cantwell, J. D., and Watt, E. W.: Extreme cardiopulmonary fitness in old age, Chest 65:357, 1974.
4. Pipes, T. V., and Wilmore, J. H.: Isokinetic vs. isotonic strength training in adult men, Med. Sci. Sports 7:262, 1975.
5. Wilmore, J. H.: Alterations in strength, body composition and anthropometric measurements consequent to a 10-week training program, Med. Sci. Sports 6:133, 1974.
6. Gwinup, G., Chelvam, R., and Steinberg, T.: Thickness of subcutaneous fat and activity of underlying muscles, Ann. Intern. Med. 74:408, 1971.
7. Clarke, H. H.: Development of muscular strength and endurance, Phys. Fitness Res. Dig. series 4, no. 1, 1974.
8. Clarke, H. H.: Strength development and motor-sports improvement, Phys. Fitness Res. Dig. series 4, no. 4, 1974.
9. Clarke, H. H.: Exercise and the knee joint, Phys. Fitness Res. Dig. series 6, no. 1, 1976.
10. Sheehan, G.: Where to put the blame for muscle pulls, Phys. Sportsmed. 4:24, 1976.
11. Wilmore, J. H., Parr, R. B., Haskell, W. L., et al.: Football pros' strengths—and CV weakness—charted, Phys. Sportsmed. 4:45, 1976.
12. Medical Times, May 1976.
13. Groom, D.: Cardiovascular observations on Tarahumara Indian Runners—the modern Spartans, Am. Heart J. 81:304, 1971.

2 / The Physiology of Exercise: Selected Aspects

This chapter discusses selected aspects of exercise physiology, emphasizing recent data on fuel homeostasis in exercise, concepts of muscle structure and function, aerobic capacity and other effects of training. We have not attempted to provide a comprehensive analysis of all aspects of exercise physiology and recommend a reference such as Astrand and Rodahl's *Textbook of Work Physiology*[1] for those who wish to study these concepts in greater depth.

FUEL CONSUMPTION DURING EXERCISE

The body can produce energy with oxygen (aerobically) or without it (anaerobically). Energy from anaerobic metabolism is produced from rupture of the terminal high-energy phosphate bond of adenosine triphosphate (ATP) to yield adenosine diphosphate (ADP) and phosphate. The energy to reconvert ADP to ATP is provided by creatine phosphate (CP), which produces energy by breaking down into creatine and phosphate, which in turn must be resynthesized. Energy to reform CP is produced from the breakdown of glycogen stored in the muscle and from the oxidation of glucose and fatty acids transported to the muscle by the bloodstream. These concepts are depicted in the following formulas:

1. $ATP \rightleftharpoons ADP + P + \text{free energy}$
2. $CP + ADP \rightleftharpoons \text{creatine} + ATP$
3. $\text{Glycogen (or glucose)} + P + ADP \rightarrow \text{lactate} + ATP$.

The disadvantages inherent in the third formula are obvious. During vigorous exercise, when the lungs and bloodstream are unable to supply the oxygen demands of the muscles, the pyruvate produced by the burning of glycogen is converted to lactic acid, which builds up in the muscle and overflows into the bloodstream. Much of the lactic acid is transported to the liver, where it is reconverted into glycogen. However, a certain amount of lactic acid accumulates in the muscle and is thought by some to contribute to premature muscle exhaustion.

Aerobic metabolism is obviously the more efficient pathway of energy production, for its yield of high-energy units is about 20 times greater than that produced through anaerobic metabolism. The formula for aerobic metabolism is:

Glycogen and free fatty acid
$$+ \: P + ADP + oxygen \rightarrow CO_2 + H_2O + ATP$$

The energy yield from fatty acids is higher than that from glucose; 1 gm of fat yields 9 k-cal of heat, while 1 gm of glucose (or protein) yields 4 k-cal of heat.

What happens during endurance exercise?[1] During the first 5–10 minutes of a long-distance run, muscle glycogen is the major fuel consumed. After 10–40 minutes of continuous exercise, the muscle uses glucose from the bloodstream. The liver contributes to blood glucose by breaking down its glycogen stores. Muscle glycogen does not contribute to blood glucose levels since muscle lacks the enzyme G-6-phosphatase needed to convert glycogen to glucose. After 60–240 minutes of exercise, the working muscle begins to oxidize fatty acid. This increased uptake of fatty acid in the physically fit person seems to decrease glucose uptake and may help to prevent hypoglycemia during extended exercise.

The intensity of exercise also plays a part in determining the fuel used for energy production. At moderate levels of exercise, energy production is approximately 50% from fat and 50% from carbohydrate. As maximum tolerance is approached, the body tends to rely on carbohydrate rather than fat, and this can pose problems since fat stores are much more plentiful than carbohydrate stores. The untrained person will quickly elevate the heart rate and approach the maximum tolerance for work, relying on limited stores of carbohydrate (glucose, glycogen), while the well-trained person, doing the same amount of work with a lower heart rate and at less than maximum tolerance, can continue to use the more plentiful fatty acid, which yields more energy per gram than does carbohydrate.

Some interesting things happen to glucose during exercise. After 90 minutes blood glucose (sugar) falls by 10–40 mg/100 ml. Fortunately, the liver can produce glucose, 75% of which comes from breakdown of glycogen and 25% from such substances as alanine (a protein subunit), lactate, pyruvate and glycerol. As exercise is prolonged, almost half the liver's glucose output comes from this manufacturing process. Hormonal changes with vigorous exercise (lowered insulin and elevated glucagon, growth hormone and catecholamine levels) contribute to the glycogenolytic and gluconeogenic responses but have not been proved essential to the exercise-stimulated hepatic glucose output.[2]

Interestingly, muscle cells take up glucose more readily during exercise, even though blood insulin levels fall. No other hormonal change during exercise seems to account for this fact, leading some to postulate that exercise itself may accomplish one function of insulin, namely, to enhance the movement of glucose across cell walls.

MUSCLE FUNCTION

The limiting factor to very strenuous work is the muscle glycogen store.[3] In trained dogs, plasma free fatty acid supplied 50–90% of energy (versus only 10% from glucose) during prolonged exercise. Such oxidation of free fatty acids spares muscle glycogen, thereby increasing endurance. In untrained dogs, mobilization of free fatty acid was inhibited during vigorous work; it is perhaps the high level of blood lactate that inhibits such mobilization, necessitating the use of muscle glycogen for fuel.

Much has been written about muscle fiber types in various athletes.[4, 5] Endurance athletes, such as long-distance runners, have more red (slow twitch) muscle fibers than white (fast twitch) fibers, which are more common in athletes engaged in anaerobic activities such as weightlifting and sprinting. Red muscle has a high capacity for breaking down glucose and glycogen for energy, the so-called aerobic metabolic process. White muscle fibers derive most of their energy from anaerobic metabolism and have the capacity to rapidly deplete their glycogen stores and to produce lactate.

The enzyme levels of both muscle fiber types can be increased with endurance training. For example, the levels of hexokinase increase more in the trained red fibers than in the white fibers, and the cytochrome c enzyme increases by 60% with training, due to both an increase in synthesis and a decrease in degradation. Because of these enzyme changes, skeletal muscle becomes more like heart muscle. Although enzyme content can be altered during endurance training, a white fiber cannot be converted to a red fiber. One group of untrained men underwent endurance training for 4 hours per week over a 5-month period; muscle biopsies showed no change in the relative percentage of red and of white muscle fibers.[6]

As white fibers cannot be changed to red fibers with training, neither can the speed of muscle contraction (or the quickness and strength of muscle response) be increased with training. Like skeletal muscle, the speed of heart muscle contraction is not increased with training.

Costill and colleagues[7] performed biopsies of the gastrocnemius muscle in 14 champion long-distance runners, 18 middle-distance runners and 19 untrained men. They found that the elite long-distance runners had 79% slow twitch fibers in the leg muscle studied, and that the slow twitch fibers had a 22% larger cross-sectional area than the fast twitch fibers. Jeff Galloway (Fig 2–1), a member of the 1972 U.S. Olympic marathon team, had the greatest percentage of slow twitch fibers in the group, an astounding 98%. The late Steve Prefontaine, with one of the highest recorded oxygen consumption rates (84 ml/kg/min), had 77% slow twitch fibers. Don Kardong, who finished 4th in the 1976 Olympic marathon, had only 53% slow twitch fibers, indicating that one can certainly be a champion runner without ideal muscle composition, which appears to be hereditary. Curiously, a predominance of fast twitch or

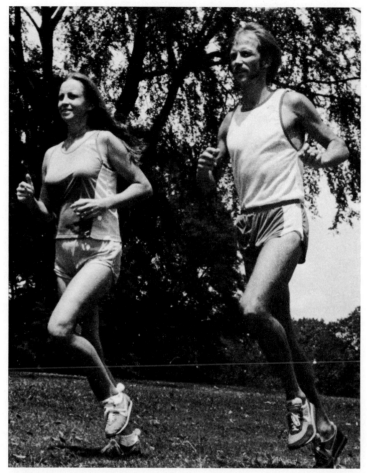

Fig 2–1.—Jeff Galloway, shown running with his wife, Barbara, had one of the highest percentages of slow twitch muscle fibers (98%) on biopsy study of elite runners.

slow twitch muscle fibers did not seem significant in a comparison of elite cyclists with their less successful peers.[8]

Costill reviewed theories of muscle exhaustion during distance running.[9] Some[2] have pointed out that lactate accumulation could interfere with muscle contraction, as the hydrogen ion competes with calcium for binding sites controlling actin-myosin interaction. Most well-trained athletes begin to accumulate lactate as they exceed 70% of their maximum oxygen uptake. Derek Clayton, who still holds the world record for the marathon, was unique in that he could work at 85–89% of his maximum capacity without accumulating lactate. It is typical of trained muscle not only to have lower lactate levels at a given level of exercise but also to have less depletion of glycogen stores and greater oxidation of free fatty acids during submaximal exercise.

It is difficult to fully explain muscle exhaustion on the basis of lactate accumulation, however, for the amount of lactic acid in the blood after a marathon race is not much higher than the baseline level. Hence, the search for other explanations continues. During intense exercise, exhaustion coincides with depletion of muscle glycogen.[4] It is unclear why such depletion should induce exhaustion, however, for other substrates (such as blood glucose and fatty acids) are available for energy production.[2] It has been shown that glycogen can be selectively depleted in the slow twitch muscle fibers of endurance athletes and also that it takes about 2 days to replenish muscle glycogen after a strenuous long-distance run.

Other attempts to explain muscle exhaustion have involved hypoglycemia, dehydration, electrolyte losses or shifts, and hyperthermia.

Muscle glycogen stores can be enhanced through the process of dietary carbohydrate "loading."[10] On a normal mixed diet, the glycogen content of the quadriceps muscle is 1.5 gm/100 gm of muscle tissue; this can provide for up to 2 hours of heavy exercise, such as marathon running. If the prerace diet is high in carbohydrate, the muscle glycogen content can be raised to 2.5 gm/100 gm of muscle. If one avoids carbohydrates for several days prior to the race, exercises to exhaustion and then loads up on carbohydrates immediately before the race, the muscle glycogen stores can exceed 4 gm/100 gm of muscle. This could provide an extra source for muscle energy and perhaps delay muscle exhaustion, if it is indeed related to muscle-glycogen depletion. We do not recommend carbohydrate loading for the average "fun runner" until the safety of this technique is established (see Chap. 9).

OXYGEN UPTAKE

Studies in young monozygotic and dizygotic twins[11] support the concept that maximum oxygen uptake is largely hereditary. However, there may be up to a 40% difference in maximum oxygen uptake in monozygotic twins when one trains and the other does not.

Two factors explain the increased maximum oxygen uptake with training:

1. The cardiac output increases because of the elevation in stroke volume.[3]
2. The arteriovenous oxygen difference widens as the working muscle is able to extract more oxygen. The latter may reflect an increase both in muscle mitochondria and in myoglobin.[12]

Even when the heart rate is lowered with propranolol, one can still reach a maximum oxygen uptake, although the maximum heart rate may be 40 beats per minute lower. This is due to the compensatory increase in stroke volume and the enhanced utilization of oxygen in the blood.[8]

The usual decline in maximum heart rate and in maximum oxygen uptake with age may be counteracted to some extent with long-term exercise. Kasch[13] did a 10-year follow-up study on men who exercised regularly and found little decline in their maximum levels, which were 36% above average in one group.

The change in maximum oxygen uptake with physical training will be influenced by both the frequency and the intensity of the training sessions. Pollock et al.[14] studied 148 normal sedentary men, aged 28–64 years, who ran for 30–45 minutes either 2, 3 or 4 times per week (groups A, B and C, respectively). Groups A and B increased their oxygen uptake by 16–17% after the 20-week training session, while the men in group C increased their maximum oxygen uptake by 22%. In another study,[15] 22 men, aged 30–45 years, were randomly assigned to 1 of 2 exercise groups. Group 1 trained for 44 minutes twice weekly at 92% of their maximum heart rate. The average exercise heart rate was 173 beats per minute. The second group exercised for 47 minutes twice a week at 80% of their maximum heart rate. The average training heart rate in this group was 161 beats per minute. After 20 weeks, the maximum oxygen uptake was 5% higher in group 1 than in group 2.

WARM-UP AND "SECOND WIND"

The benefits of warm-up exercise on performance are inconclusive. Karpovich et al.[16] found that a warm-up did not significantly improve finish times in the 440-yard dash. On the other hand, Watt et al.[17] found that the oxygen uptake level and exercise heart rate were significantly higher in 8 men during an exhaustive run following a warm-up than they were without a warm-up. A recent treadmill study of California firemen[18] suggested that ischemic electrocardiographic changes could frequently be produced in apparently healthy men when the treadmill protocol did not include a warm-up phase. It would seem prudent always to include a warm-up period before endurance exercise if for no other reason than to try to reduce the frequency of musculotendinous injuries.

Although athletes repeatedly refer to the concept of a "second wind," the physiological explanation of such a phenomenon has been elusive. Shephard[19] found no significant changes in heart rates or in respiratory rates of athletes at the time they experienced second wind. Moreover, the latter occurred anywhere from 2 to 18 minutes in a 20-minute treadmill test. Shephard lists several possibilities to account for the subjective sensation:

1. At some point in a running event the athlete could surpass his or her anaerobic threshold, with resulting lactate production and hyperventilation from metabolic acidosis. The runner might unconsciously alter his pace slightly, slipping back under the anaerobic threshold (which may vary between 50 and 80% of the maximum exercise tolerance).

2. There may be initial difficulty in perfusing an active muscle that is developing over 15% of its maximum voluntary force. This could produce temporary muscle fatigue that is relieved when the exercise-induced blood pressure rise facilitates muscle perfusion.

3. The initial response to exercise is transient vasoconstriction of the muscle's arteries; this may last from 30–60 seconds and might temporarily increase lactate production in the muscle. This situation is quickly remedied when accumulations of potassium ion and carbon dioxide, along with reduction in available oxygen, stimulate vasodilation.

Other considerations include lack of an adequate warm-up, intercostal muscle fatigue and psychological factors.

VIGOROUS EXERCISE AND CORONARY ARTERY DIAMETER

Animal studies[20] suggest that coronary artery diameters increase in response to vigorous exercise. The case report of lifelong distance runner Clarence DeMar,[21] as well as coronary arteriograms in several distance-running patients who had chest pain or ventricular arrhythmias, supports this theory. A recent report from Johns Hopkins[22] of 145 autopsies on persons with normal postmortem coronary angiograms showed a direct linear relationship between the heart weight and the cube of the normal coronary arterial diameter. In other words, normal coronary arteries "enlarge their caliber by at least the cube of the diameter proportionate to increase in heart size." The required blood flow volume by the hard-working myocardium seems to determine the size of the coronary arteries. This confirms the statement by Drs. Paul Wood and C. V. Harrison 30 years ago that "the size of the coronary arteries varies directly with the heart weight in normal and hypertrophied hearts irrespective of the cause of hypertrophy."[23]

The long-distance runner, swimmer or cyclist may not only be developing the athlete's hypertrophied ventricle, but may also be enlarging the diameter of the coronary arteries.

THE ATHLETE'S SLOW PULSE

Paul Dudley White was among the first to observe marked bradycardia in a distance runner whose resting heart rate was 37 beats per minute.[24] Electrocardiograms in cyclists[25] and marathon runners[26, 27] have shown resting heart rates as low as

44 beats per minute. In Chapter 3 we describe 2 male amateur runners with resting heart rates of 28 and 31, and a marathoner-nurse whose resting rate is 37 beats per minute.

Bradycardia in athletes has generally been attributed to increased vagal tone and decreased sympathetic influence. Frick et al.,[28] using atropine and propranolol to induce parasympathetic and β-adrenergic receptor blockage, found that resting bradycardia was due to parasympathetic inhibition, while the reduced heart rate during exertion indicated decreased sympathetic drive. Further evidence supporting the role of increased vagal tone was presented by Herrlich et al.,[29] who found higher acetylcholine levels in the atria of rats that were trained physically. Supportive evidence for reduced sympathetic drive is the finding of lower catecholamine levels in the plasma of physically trained, compared to untrained, persons.[30]

It is interesting that some premier distance runners, such as Jim Ryun, have relatively high resting pulse rates (64–76 beats per minute in Ryun's case)[31] while a jogger, like one of those mentioned above, may have extreme bradycardia. There is undoubtedly a great deal of individual variation, the precise mechanism of which is unclear. Transient atrioventricular dissociation and Wenckebach atrioventricular block are occasionally seen in the electrocardiograms of endurance athletes[32, 33] and probably reflect the increase in vagal tone.

REFERENCES
1. Astrand, P., and Rodahl, K.: *Textbook of Work Physiology* (2d ed.; New York: McGraw-Hill Book Co., 1977).
2. Felig, P., and Wahren, J.: Fuel homeostasis in exercise, N. Engl. J. Med. 293:1078, 1975.
3. Paul, P., and Holmes, W. L.: Free fatty acid and glucose metabolism during increased energy expenditure and after training, Med. Sci. Sports 7:176, 1975.
4. Holloszy, J. O.: Adaptations of muscular tissue to training, Prog. Cardiovasc. Dis. 18:445, 1976.
5. Costill, D.: Championship material, Runner's World, April, 1974, p. 26.
6. Gollnick, P. D., Armstrong, R. B., Saltin, B., et al.: Effect of training on enzyme activity and fiber composition of human skeletal muscle, J. Appl. Physiol. 34:107, 1973.

7. Costill, D. L., Fink, W. J., and Pollock, M. L.: Muscle fiber composition and enzyme activities of elite distance runners, Med. Sci. Sports 8:96, 1976.

8. Burke, E. R., Cerny, F., Costill, D., et al.: Characteristics of skeletal muscle in competitive cyclists, Med. Sci. Sports 9:109, 1977.

9. Costill, D. L.: Muscular exhaustion during distance running, Phys. Sports Med. 2:36, 1974.

10. Astrand, P. O.: The physiology of maximal performance, Mod. Med., June 26, 1972, p. 50.

11. Bar-Or, O.: Predicting athletic performance, Phys. Sports Med. 3: 81, 1975.

12. Holloszy, J. O.: Adaptation of skeletal muscle to endurance exercise, Med. Sci. Sports 7:155, 1975.

13. Kasch, F. W.: The effects of exercise on the aging process, Phys. Sports Med. 4:64, 1976.

14. Pollock, M., Miller, H., and Linnerud, A. C.: Benefits of regularity, Runner's World, May, 1974, p. 21.

15. Pollock, M. L., Broida, J., Kendrick, Z., et al.: Effects of training two days per week at different intensities on middle-aged men, Med. Sci. Sports 4:192, 1972.

16. Karpovich, P. V., and Hale, C. J.: Effect of warm-up upon physical performance, J.A.M.A. 163:1117, 1956.

17. Watt, E. W., and Hodgson, J. L.: The effect of warm-up on total oxygen cost of a short treadmill run to exhaustion, Ergonomics 18:397, 1975.

18. Barnard, R. J., MacAlpin, R., Kattus, A. A., et al.: Ischemic response to sudden strenuous exercise in healthy men, Circulation 48:936, 1973.

19. Shephard, R. J.: What causes second wind? Phys. Sports Med. 2: 37, 1974.

20. Froelicher, V. F.: Animal studies of effect of chronic exercise on the heart and atherosclerosis: A review, Am. Heart J. 84:496, 1972.

21. Currens, J. H., and White, P. D.: Half a century of running: Clinical, physiological and autopsy findings in the case of Clarence DeMar ("Mr. Marathon"), N. Engl. J. Med. 265:988, 1961.

22. Hutchins, G. M., Bulkley, B. H., Miner, M. M., et al.: Correlations of age and heart weight with tortuosity and caliber of normal human coronary arteries, Am. Heart J. 94:196, 1977.

23. Harrison, C. V., and Wood, P.: Hypertensive and ischemic heart disease: A comparative clinical and pathological study, Br. Heart J. 11:205, 1949.

24. White, P. D., and Donovan, H.: *Hearts: Their Long-Term Follow-up* (Philadelphia: W. B. Saunders Co., 1967).

25. Van Ganse, W., Versee, L., Eylenbosch, W., et al.: The electrocardiogram of athletes, Br. Heart J. 32:160, 1970.

26. Nakamoto, K.: Electrocardiograms of 25 marathon runners before and after 100 meter dash, Japanese Circ. J. 33:105, 1969.
27. Smith, W. G., Cullen, K. J., and Thorburn, I. L.: Electrocardiograms of marathon runners in 1962 Commonwealth Games, Br. Heart J. 26:469, 1964.
28. Frick, M. H., Elovainio, R. O., and Somer, T.: The mechanism of bradycardia evoked by physical training, Cardiology 51:46, 1967.
29. Herrlich, H. C., Raab, W., and Gigee, W.: Influence of muscular training and of catecholamines on cardiac acetylcholine and cholinesterase, Arch. Int. Pharmacodyn. Ther. 129:201, 1960.
30. Simpson, M. T., Hames, C. G., Olewine, D. A., et al.: Physical activity, catecholamines, and platelet stickiness, Conference on Preventive Myocardiology of the American College of Cardiology, Stowe, Vt., June 1970.
31. Daniels, J. T.: Running with Jim Ryun: A five-year study, Phys. Sports Med. 2:62, 1974.
32. Lichtman, J., O'Rourke, R., Klein, A., et al.: Electrocardiogram of the athlete, Arch. Intern. Med. 132:763, 1973.
33. Meytes, I., Kaplinsky, E., Yahini, J. H., et al.: Wenckebach A-V block: A frequent feature following heavy physical training, Am. Heart J. 90:426, 1975.

3 / Testing the Athlete

Today it is possible to test the various aspects of an athlete's physical fitness in order to predict his or her potential, assess the response to a physical training program or to measure the degree of rehabilitation.

In chapter 2 we discussed muscle biopsy data and techniques; these could constitute one parameter to determine the ideal sport for an aspiring athlete. For example, a predominance of red muscle (slow-twitch) fibers in a 13-year-old could be one factor pointing him toward an endurance sport such as distance running—a sport best suited to his physiology. Another finding that might steer him toward this type of sport would be an unusually high (> 65 ml/kg/min) oxygen uptake on treadmill stress testing.

THE PREPARTICIPATION MEDICAL EVALUATION

Before participating in competitive sports, prospective athletes should have a complete medical history taken and a thorough physical examination performed. Those with a family history of cardiovascular disease should have serum cholesterol, triglyceride, and high-density lipoprotein levels measured. Resting ECGs and chest x-rays should be obtained when there is a history of any cardiac disorder or if the physical examination reveals any significant abnormality. Noninvasive studies such as exercise stress testing and echocardiography are useful in selected instances (see Chap. 5) but are not recommended as routine screening measures. Any abnormalities in standard laboratory tests (blood count, urinalysis) should be referred to the family physician or appropriate specialist for investigation before the athlete begins practice sessions.

BODY COMPOSITION ANALYSIS

Several indirect methods — x-rays of subcutaneous fat, measurement of body density and total body water, and the use of fat-soluble indicators — can be used to estimate the ratio of lean body mass to body fat. A useful technique in office practice, or for mass screening, is the measuring of skinfold thickness by constant-tension skinfold calipers (Fig. 3–1). Such determinations, checking thickness at 10 body sites, have cor-

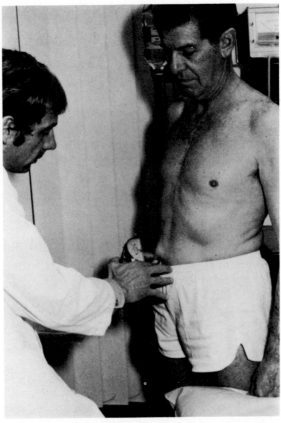

Fig 3–1. — Measurement of body composition analysis, using the skinfold caliper technique.

related well with body-fat calculations obtained by other methods, such as underwater weighing.

We studied a large-framed professional baseball pitcher who was interested in knowing his ideal body weight. He thought that by reaching this standard, his pitching would improve. He was 6′ 1″ tall and weighed 210 pounds. By measuring 10 skinfold sites, we calculated his body fat at 19%. We recommended that he reduce his weight to 195 pounds, at which level we would repeat the measurement. Because this pitcher was traded shortly after our evaluation, there was no medical followup. However, he has been a good relief pitcher for 2 years.

If the percentage of body fat is greater than the upper normal limit of 14% (17% for women), we recommend either additional weight loss or weight training to increase lean-muscle mass.

STRENGTH, POWER AND ENDURANCE

Previously, strength has been measured by leg and grip dynamometers and by the one-REM technique (using the curl, bench press or other muscle group exercises). Recent methods use Cybex isokinetic equipment (Fig 3–2, A), which can measure muscle strength, endurance and power. For example, Figure 3–2, B shows the relative strength in the quadriceps muscle group in the right leg versus the hamstring strength; Figure 3–2, C shows the relative power (or the rate of work) in the same muscle groups. One can also measure quadriceps endurance (number of repetitions to 50% fatigue — when the testing graph scale is decreased 50%), which, in the case depicted here, takes 28 repetitions. Comparative tests of the same muscle groups in the right and left legs can then be done.

FLEXIBILITY

Different types of activities require varying amounts of flexibility. Some activities, such as distance running, reduce flexibility, especiallly in the lower back and legs. Good flexibility

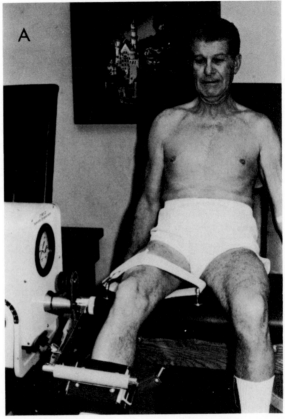

Fig 3–2.— A, testing muscle strength, power and endurance on the Cybex device. *(Continued)*

should always be emphasized by coaches, trainers and team physicians (Fig 3–3).

Range of joint motion can be measured with Cybex equipment.[1] The Leighton Flexometer can test the movements of at least 30 joints. Simpler tests for flexibility include the "sit-and-reach" test and the "back hyperextension" test. In the former, one measures the distance the sitting subject can reach beyond the tip of the toes. In the latter, the subject is prone and, upon command, hyperextends the back. The exam-

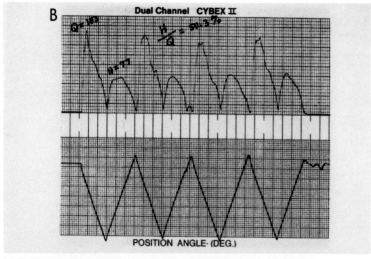

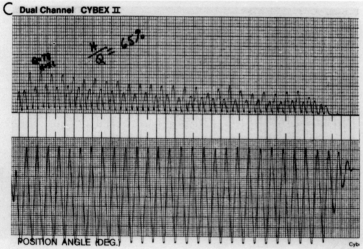

Fig 3–2 (cont.) – B, relative quadriceps : hamstring strength in the right leg of a subject. **C,** relative power in the same muscle groups in **B.**

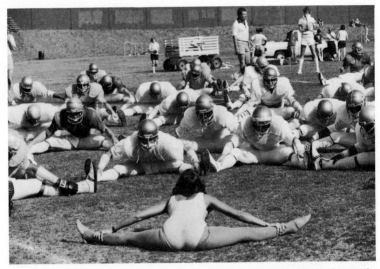

Fig 3–3. — Fitness instructor leads Georgia Tech football players in stretching exercises to improve their flexibility. (*Atlanta Journal-Constitution* photo; used by permission.)

iner multiplies the distance between the floor and the sternal notch by 100 and divides by the seated sternal notch height.

In studies on 139 New York Jet football players, Nicholas[2] emphasized the importance of flexibility. He considered players to be "tight-jointed" if they:

- were unable to touch the floor with their palms (bending from the waist, with the knees kept straight)
- were unable to sit comfortably in the lotus position
- had less than a 20-degree hyperextension of the knees while lying prone on a table with the legs hanging over the end
- were unable to position their feet at 180 degrees while standing with the knees flexed 15–30 degrees
- had no upper arm laxity on shoulder flexion, elbow hyperextension and forearm hypersupination.

He found that 50 of the 139 players (36%) were tight-jointed. These athletes were susceptible to muscle pulls or tears, while the loose-jointed athletes were more likely to rupture

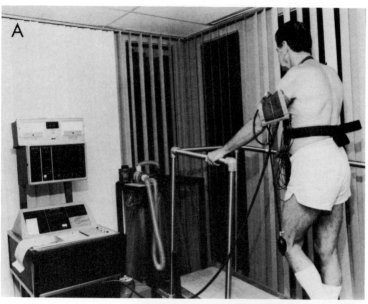

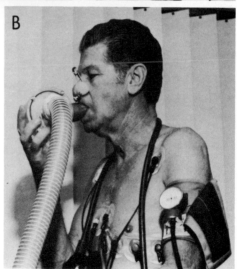

Fig 3–4. — Exercise testing (treadmill technique), with oxygen-uptake analysis and 12-lead ECG monitoring.

ligaments. Nicholas concluded that "tight" athletes should do stretching exercises, while "loose" athletes should concentrate on developing power with resistive exercises. Godshall[3] did not find the same correlation between loose-jointedness and major injuries in high-school football players.

EXERCISE STRESS TESTING

The most precise way to determine heart and lung fitness is to measure oxygen consumption at the maximum workload on a bicycle ergometer or a treadmill (Fig 3–4, A and B). By plotting the oxygen uptake on the ordinant, and the subject's age on the abscissa, one can get a pinpoint classification of fitness (Fig 3–5).

The exercise test has other uses. One can have a normal resting ECG (Fig 3–6) and develop ST-segment depression

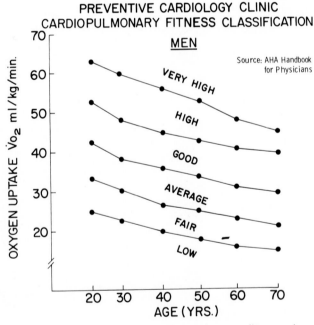

Fig 3–5.—Classification of cardiorespiratory fitness, based on oxygen-uptake analysis.

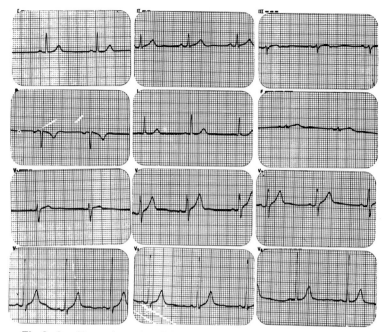

Fig 3–6. — Normal resting ECG in a subject with 3-vessel coronary heart disease.

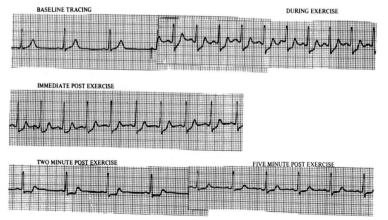

Fig 3–7. — An abnormal exercise ECG in the subject described in Fig 3–6.

during exercise (Fig 3–7), which is usually a clue to underlying coronary heart disease (severe in the case depicted). With more and more middle-aged people taking up vigorous exercise such as jogging, it is important to identify those who might be risking cardiac catastrophe during such activity. A middle-aged professor with a past history of a mild coronary attack had been jogging a mile or so several days per week

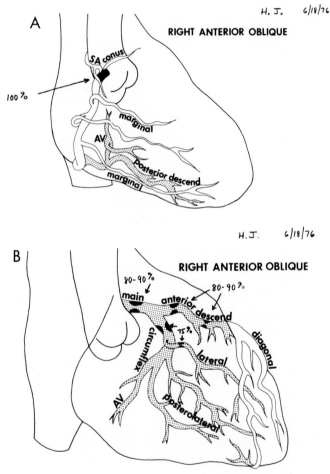

Fig 3–8. — Extensive coronary disease in an asymptomatic middle-aged jogger with prior history of a coronary event.

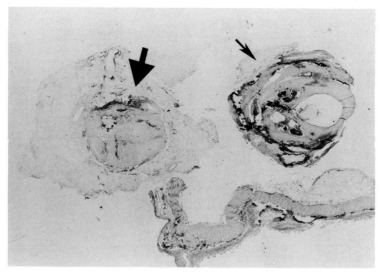

Fig 3–9.—Extensive coronary disease at autopsy in a 53-year-old physician who collapsed after jogging 1 mile.

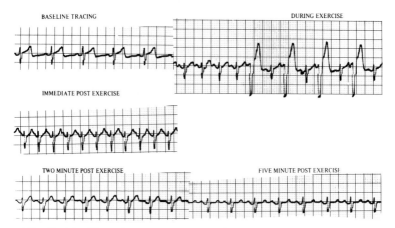

Fig 3–10.—Transient ventricular bigeminy, with normal ST segments, in a 41-year-old man.

with no symptoms. A friend suggested that he have an exercise stress test, which showed marked ST-segment depression. Coronary arteriograms showed extensive blockage of all coronary arteries (Fig 3–8, A and B). Even though he was asymptomatic, the man was advised to undergo coronary artery bypass surgery. His postoperative exercise test is now normal. A physician of similar age, who was not so fortunate, collapsed after jogging and could not be revived. The autopsy

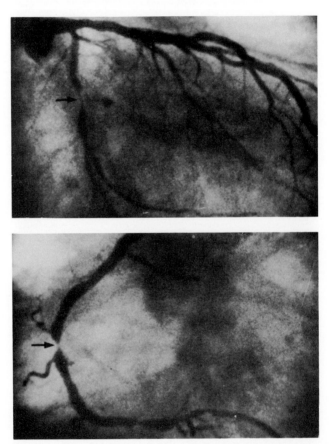

Fig 3–11.—Near-total occlusion of the left circumflex coronary *(top)* and mid-right coronary arteries in the subject described in Figure 3–9.

revealed extensive coronary disease (Fig 3–9) similar to that of the previously mentioned professor.

The exercise ECG is not a perfect diagnostic tool, for up to 25–35% of those with underlying coronary disease have normal stress tests. An example is a 41-year-old man whose exercise test was unremarkable except for transient ventricular bigeminy during exercise (Fig 3–10). He was seen again 6 weeks later because of severe chest pain and underwent coronary arteriography, which revealed near-total occlusion of the left circumflex coronary artery and of the mid-right coronary vessel (Fig 3–11). False positive tests can likewise pose problems in young athletes. We saw a former rugby player who complained of chest pain atypical for angina pectoris. His exercise ECG (Fig 3–12) was worrisome, even though the ST-T change when the patient stood raised the possibility of a false positive response. The patient wished to maintain a vigorous lifestyle, jogging and traveling extensively. Coronary arteriography revealed normal vasculature, and he was cleared for such activities.

The exercise ECG may be useful to assess the relationship of ventricular premature beats to exercise, and vice versa. A pilot wished to jog, but was concerned by palpitations. These were found to result from ventricular parasystole (Fig 3–13); there was no other evidence to suggest underlying heart disease. His rhythm was perfectly regular during and immediately following maximal exercise testing, and he was cleared for a home jogging program. The opposite situation was noted in a 50-year-old man who had marked ventricular irritabilities on exercise testing (Fig 3–14). He was treated with antiarrhythmic drugs and, when his rhythm stabilized, was referred to our medically supervised gym program, where his heart beat could be closely monitored by "instant electrocardiography," using printout paddle electrodes from the defibrillator (Fig 3–15).

Occasionally, subjects exhibit hypertensive responses to exercise testing. Such patients may have labile hypertension and should have a comprehensive coronary risk-factor workup, followed by close monitoring of blood pressure.

In over 1500 exercise tests of apparently healthy people, we

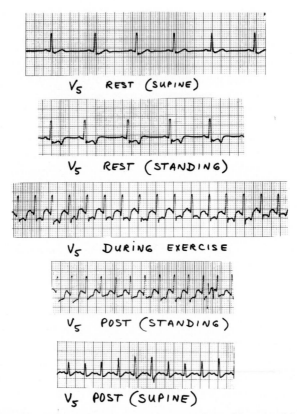

Fig 3–12.—False-positive exercise test in a 33-year-old former rugby player.

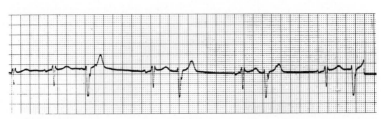

Fig 3–13.—Ventricular parasystole in a pilot with an otherwise normal cardiovascular examination.

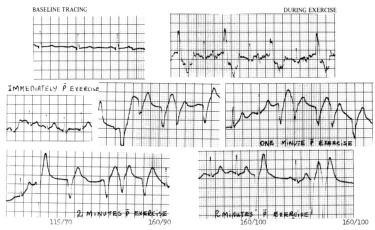

Fig 3–14.—Marked ventricular irritability during exercise in a 50-year-old man.

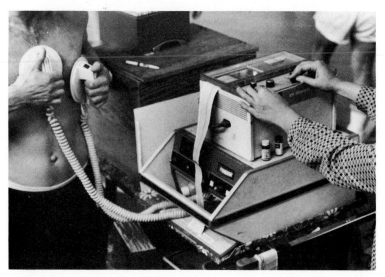

Fig 3–15.—Instant ECG technique for rhythm analysis, used in the cardiac rehabilitation program at Georgia Baptist Hospital.

have seen some interesting cases. The record time on our treadmill test (22 minutes, using the Bruce technique) belongs to Gayle Barron (Fig 3–16), a 33-year-old former University of Georgia cheerleader who began jogging in college. She finished among the top four women in the 1975 and 1976 Boston Marathons and won the women's division race in 1978 (in 2:

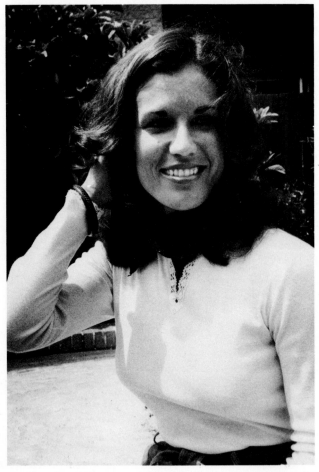

Fig 3–16. — Gayle Barron, world-class distance runner, and winner of the 1978 Boston Marathon (women's division), who completed 22 minutes of the Bruce treadmill test. (Courtesy of Bill Wilson.)

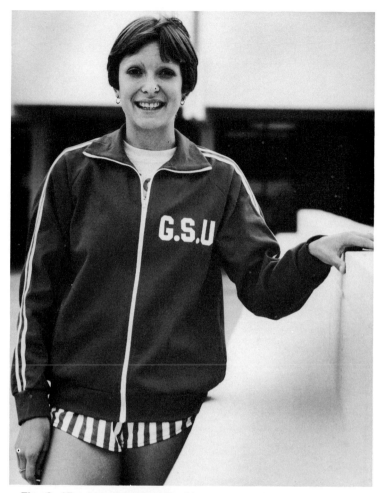

Fig 3–17. — Lisa Lorrain Hoskins, a marathon-running nurse-graduate student. (Courtesy of George Clark.)

44:52). She also placed third in the 1976 International Women's Marathon in Waldneil, Germany. Lisa Lorrain Hoskins (Fig 3–17), a 24-year-old registered nurse who is 5' 4" tall, took up distance running when her weight rose to 140 pounds. Her weight dropped to 115 pounds, and she placed 9th among

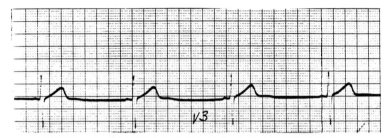

Fig 3–18. — Resting heart rate of 37 beats per minute in Lisa Lorrain Hoskins.

women in the 1976 Boston Marathon and captured the women's division of the 1976 Peach Bowl Marathon, covering the distance in 2:51. Lisa's resting heart rate (Fig 3–18) is 37 beats per minute, the slowest we have seen in a female athlete.

The slowest resting pulse we have seen was in 40-year-old

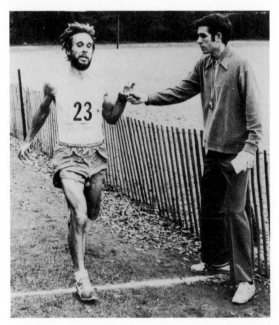

Fig 3–19. — 40-year-old Charles Feaux, a veteran runner who covers up to 100 miles per week. (Reprinted, with permission, from Phys. Sportsmed.)

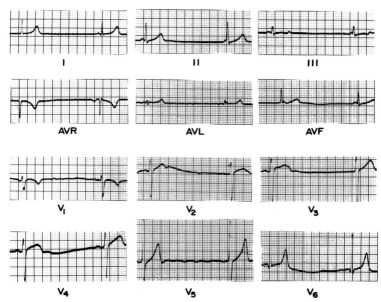

Fig 3–20. — Resting heart rate of 28 beats per minute in Charles Feaux. (Reprinted, with permission, from Phys. Sportsmed.)

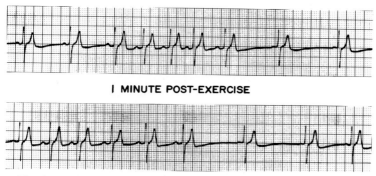

I MINUTE POST-EXERCISE

Fig 3–21. — Remarkable pulse recovery 1 minute after maximal exercise test in subject described in Figures 3–19 and 3–20. (Reprinted, with permission, from Phys. Sportsmed.)

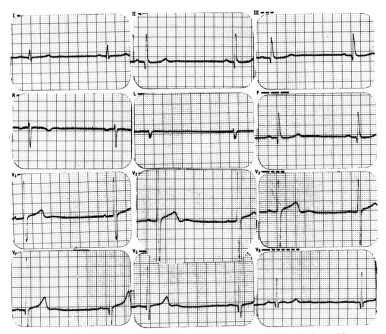

Fig 3–22. — Resting pulse rate of 31 beats per minute in a 43-year-old pilot who jogs 12–15 miles per week. (Reprinted, with permission, from Phys. Sportsmed.)

Charles Feaux (Fig 3–19), a veteran distance runner who runs up to 100 miles per week. His pulse rate was 28 beats per minute (Fig 3–20). His maximum response to 17 minutes on the Bruce test was 155 beats per minute; the maximum oxygen uptake was 57.9 ml/kg/min. One minute after stopping exercise, his heart rate was 44 beats per minute (Fig 3–21).

Another extremely slow pulse rate was seen in a 43-year-old commercial pilot who had been jogging for 7 years and had gradually worked up to his present level of a 3-mile jog 4 to 5 times per week. His resting pulse was 31 beats per minute (Fig 3–22).

REFERENCES

1. Cybex II Testing Protocol, Lumex, Inc., 1975.
2. Nicholas, J. A.: Injuries to knee ligaments: relationship to looseness and tightness in football players, J.A.M.A. 212:2236, 1970.

3. Godshall, R. W.: The predictability of athletic injuries: an eight-year study, J. Sports Med. 3:50, 1975.
4. Clarke, H. H. (ed.): Joint and body range of movement, Phys. Fitness Res. Dig., series 5, no. 4, 1975.
5. Fortuin, N. J., and Weiss, J. L.: Exercise stress testing, Circulation 56:699, 1977.

4 / General Medical Problems in Sports

A wide spectrum of medical problems may be encountered by the sports-oriented physician. While most of the problems, such as upper respiratory infections, will be mundane, a few will challenge the physician's diagnostic capabilities, as evidenced by the recent tragic death of a college football player from leptospirosis, which had caused high fever and cardiac failure.

In this chapter we will discuss some of the more common medical problems that a team physician is called upon to evaluate. Cardiovascular conditions will be considered in Chapter 5.

THE HEAD

Eyes

Conjunctivitis is a common eye problem. It is usually of bacterial, viral or allergic etiology, or it may be caused by foreign bodies, chemicals and other irritants. The bacterial variety is the most common and is usually a self-limited problem, clearing in 10–14 days. An appropriate antibiotic ointment or drops based on culture of the discharge usually clears the condition in 2 or 3 days. In viral conjunctivitis the ocular discharge is usually watery rather than purulent; this condition is also self-limited, clearing in 1–3 weeks. Antibiotics are ineffective in treating the virus but might reduce the incidence of secondary bacterial infection.

The athlete may occasionally complain of burning or irritation of the eyes, with no evidence of inflammation on examination. Eyedrops, such as Visine or Murine, may provide symptomatic relief.

Foreign particles are removed by everting the upper eyelid and irrigating the eye gently with sterile water. An ophthalmologist should be consulted if the foreign body remains embedded. The athlete should be carefully questioned about possible symptoms of retinal detachment, such as light flashes or black floaters. If either of these symptoms is present, a thorough examination by an ophthalmologist should be promptly arranged.

A sty indicates infection of the meibomian glands, Moll's glands or the glands of Zeis. *Staphylococcus aureus* is often the offending organism. Warm compresses are applied for 15 minutes, 4 times daily, and antibiotic drops are instilled after obtaining a culture of the lesion. Occasionally, it is necessary to incise a large meibomian gland abscess. A sterile granulomatous inflammation of the meibomian gland is called a chalazion. It differs from a sty in that the lesion is not acutely inflamed, does not respond well to antibiotics and may need to be excised if it interferes with vision.

Ears, Nose and Throat

A sensation of fullness in the ears may indicate a cerumen plug. Gentle irrigation with lukewarm water usually produces satisfactory relief. Cerumenex drops may help to dislodge impacted cerumen. With the head tilted sideways 45 degrees, the ear canal is filled with Cerumenex drops. A cotton plug is inserted and left in place for 15–30 minutes. The ear is then gently flushed with lukewarm water, using a soft rubber syringe and avoiding excessive pressure. A second application may be necessary for excessively hard impactions. The drops should not be used in individuals with a history of a perforated eardrum or of general allergic reactions. If the drug comes in contact with the skin, it should be promptly washed off with soap and water.

For otitis externa, cortisporin (4 drops q.i.d. in the affected ear) is the drug of choice, as it kills a wide variety of gram-positive and gram-negative organisms. The steroid component in the drops helps to relieve itching and inflammation.

For otitis media, ampicillin (250 mg q.i.d.) is the most frequently prescribed drug. Amoxicillin (Larotid) has an antibacterial spectrum similar to that of ampicillin but is better absorbed from the gastrointestinal tract, providing higher serum levels at comparable doses. This benefit must be weighed against the cost of the drug. Erythromycin can be used in those patients allergic to penicillin.

The common cold and sinus congestion are ubiquitous in sports medicine. A yellowish postnasal drip should be cultured, as should a sore throat, and appropriate antibiotics utilized if the culture is positive. A variety of antihistamines and decongestants, such as Dimetapp, Actifed and Ornade, are commonly used and may provide some symptomatic relief, although well-controlled studies as to overall efficacy are generally lacking. It is best for the athlete to avoid these drugs within 4–6 hours of a game, as they may induce drowsiness, nervousness and visual disturbances.

If the athlete complaining of a "cold" has yellowish sputum, and if the lungs are clear on auscultation, tetracycline or ampicillin is usually prescribed, pending the culture results. If the tonsils are purulent, an injection of benzathine penicillin is given or oral penicillin is started, pending the culture report.

Many athletes take vitamin C, hoping to reduce the frequency or intensity of colds. Studies have not consistently shown this to be efficacious. However, there is no harm in taking 500 mg of the vitamin every day if the athlete thinks it might be helpful in his individual case.

THE CHEST

Tracheobronchitis and Pneumonia

Tracheobronchitis and pneumonia are infrequently found in the athlete. The diagnosis is usually easily established with a careful history and physical examination, sputum gram stains and cultures, and chest x-ray findings. A 7- to 10-day course of the appropriate antibiotic, in conjunction with rest and ample fluid intake, usually results in prompt cure. The athlete should be kept out of competition until the chest x-ray shows that the infiltrate has cleared.

Asthma

Five medal winners in the 1972 Summer Olympics were asthmatic, proving that such individuals need not be rendered ineffective in sports.

Exercise-induced asthma is a well-recognized entity, the mechanism of which is not clear. Ferguson et al.[1] thought that it could be partly explained by hyperventilation, pointing out that postexercise hyperventilation can lead to hypocapnia and consequent bronchospasm. The latter can be reversed by adding CO_2 to the inspired air.

Katz[2] indicates that exercise-induced asthma does not seem related to blood gas abnormalities or to acidosis. Serotonin is not implicated, but bradykinin and slow-reacting substance are possible culprits. Some children with this disorder had ventilation-perfusion abnormalities even before exercise.

In an excellent overview, Shephard[3] discusses the nuances of exercise-induced bronchospasm (EIB), including studies proving and disproving various theories on pathogenesis (reflex stimulation of vagal pathways, increase in lactate or hydrogen ion concentration, hypoxemia, hypocapnia, hyperventilation, humoral responses, imbalance of α- and β-adrenergic stimulation, and nonspecific stress factors). Recent research has looked at the possible role of mediators like slow-reacting substances, bradykinin, and the prostaglandins. Prostaglandin F_2 is a bronchoconstrictor, while prostaglandin E is a bronchodilator. Perhaps an imbalance of these effects induces EIB. It seems unlikely that any one mechanism can explain all instances of exercise-induced asthma. As Shephard concludes:

> At different times, the spasm is probably attributable to the vagal reflex arc, alterations of sympathetic balance, prostaglandin release, and sensitization of the mast cell. The final common path is the smooth muscle of the airways. This contracts in response to an increased concentration of cyclic guanosine monophosphate (cGMP) and relaxes in response to an increase in cyclic adenosine monophosphate (cAMP).[3]

The principal therapy in asthma involves agents that increase the effective level of cyclic AMP, which dilates smooth muscle and keeps mast cells and basophile cells from releasing histamine and slow-reacting substance. Adrenergic compounds, such as ephedrine, increase cyclic AMP formation. Aminophylline interferes with phosphodiesterase, the enzyme involved in the metabolism of cyclic AMP. Cromolyn sodium, an effective preventer of asthmatic attacks, also inhibits phosphodiesterase and prevents the mast cells from releasing their chemical mediators. Those subject to exercise-induced asthma may also be given a selective B_2 sympathomimetic drug, such as Salbutamol, prior to exercise.

Bierman et al.[4] compared ephedrine sulfate (25 mg), anhydrous theophylline (130 mg) and hydroxyzine hydrochloride (10 mg) for the relief of exercise-induced asthma. Theophylline was the most effective, while hydroxyzine was a distant second. Ephedrine had no effect. All three drugs in combination were more effective than was theophylline alone.

Cromolyn sodium (Aarane, Intal) is inhaled prior to exercise and can be taken 4 times daily. Terbutaline (Brethine), which selectively stimulates the β_2 adrenergic receptor in bronchial smooth muscle, is taken orally. The starting dose, 2.5 mg 3 times daily, can be doubled if necessary. Side effects, such as nervousness and tremor, may be noted initially. The AMA Committee on Medical Aspects of Sports has summarized° various drugs used for exercise-induced asthma (Table 4–1).

TABLE 4–1.—DRUGS FOR EXERCISE-INDUCED ASTHMA

DRUG	DOSE	ROUTE	WHEN TO GIVE (MIN BEFORE EXERCISE)
Terbutaline	5 mg (over age 12)	Oral	60
Cromolyn sodium°	20 mg	Inhalation	5–20
Theophylline + ephedrine°	½ tab (under age 10) 1 tab (over age 10)	Oral	60
Metaproterenol	20 mg	Oral or inhalation	60
Isoproterenol	14 mEq/aerosol	Inhalation	5–30

°Only cromolyn sodium and theophylline are permissible at international competitions.

' °Pamphlet OP-14, obtainable from the American Medical Association, 535 N. Dearborn, Chicago, Ill. 60610.

High-Altitude Pulmonary Edema

High-altitude pulmonary edema[5-7] (HAPE) is a problem in mountaineers, occasionally in skiers, and infrequently in distance runners who train in this environment. The initial symptoms are often similar to those in acute mountain sickness — fatigue, headache, weakness, nausea, anorexia and giddiness. This is followed by dyspnea, dry cough, substernal chest pain and eventually the production of pink, frothy sputum.

The syndrome may occur at altitudes as low as 8,000 feet. It sometimes develops during first exposure to high altitude but more often is seen in persons acclimatized to high altitude who spend several days or weeks at sea level and then reascend.

Physiological features of HAPE are: (1) increased pulmonary artery pressure and pulmonary vascular resistance, (2) normal pulmonary capillary wedge pressure, (3) hypoxemia, not corrected with 100% oxygen, and (4) normal or decreased cardiac output. Nonuniform arteriolar vasoconstriction in some lung fields, with local hyperperfusion of others, is suspected. It may be that small preterminal arterioles, which arise at right angles from small and medium-sized pulmonary arteries and empty into the pulmonary capillary bed, transport blood during arteriolar vasoconstriction, bypassing gas exchange and creating a right-to-left shunt. This might explain why 100% oxygen does not correct the hypoxemia. Widespread intravascular fibrin thrombi have been observed in some, but not all, cases of HAPE.

The mechanisms involved are not completely clear. The central nervous system symptoms have been attributed to edema of brain tissue; acetazolamide has therefore been used as a preventive measure before or during ascent. This drug increases cerebral blood flow but decreases cerebrospinal fluid production and pressure. In addition, it increases hydrogen-ion concentration in cerebrospinal fluid.

Symptoms of mild altitude sickness can be treated with aspirin and compazine. Pulmonary edema is treated with oxygen, morphine, furosemide, aminophylline, and descent to lower altitude. Digitalis preparations are usually not used.

GASTROINTESTINAL PROBLEMS

Diarrhea

We have occasionally encountered severe diarrhea in athletes, such as one of the catchers for the Atlanta Braves who had 8 or 9 loose stools prior to a game. Lomotil (2.5–5.0 mg every 6 hours) is usually effective. If diarrhea persists, the stool should be cultured and one of the following administered:

1. Donnagel-PG: ½ oz every 4 hours
2. Paregoric: 1 teaspoonful every 3–4 hours
3. Tincture of opium: 10 drops in water every 3–4 hours.

An occasional distance runner may be bothered by postrace diarrhea.[8] If lactose intake was increased in the prerace meal (e.g., milk, ice cream) diarrhea could indicate a deficiency in intestinal lactase. Other possible causes include an increase in adenyl cyclase in the intestinal cells, which could produce a secretory diarrhea, and psychological factors.

Functional Gastrointestinal Symptoms

Functional gastrointestinal symptoms, such as abdominal fullness and epigastric burning, seem more prevalent in the early part of a sports season. Most of these can be treated with routine medical measures such as simple reassurance, antacids or antiflatulents.

Viral Hepatitis

Considerable advances have been made in identifying hepatitis B antigen (Australia antigen, surface antigen, core antigen, Dane particles). The athlete infected with this virus should refrain from exercise until liver function tests have returned to normal and the liver is no longer tender on palpation. Electron-microscopy studies of stool have recently identified particles that may be hepatitis A (short-incubation) virus. Teammates of a player with hepatitis A should receive γ-globulin injections within 1–2 weeks of exposure. Gamma globulin containing high antibody titers to the surface antigen of hepatitis B may reduce the risk of this disease in close contacts of infected patients.

Hepatitis may also be caused by the Epstein-Barr virus (in

infectious mononucleosis) and cytomegalic inclusion disease. The latter illness may mimic infectious mononucleosis, except for the absence of cervical adenopathy and heterophil positivity.

GENITOURINARY SYSTEM

Albuminuria, Hematuria, Myoglobinuria[9, 10]

Functional albuminuria has been noted in athletes since at least 1907, as have hematuria and cylinduria. These conditions generally disappear within hours or days after exercise and were initially thought to be benign, perhaps a reflection of transient decreased renal blood flow or a sudden increase in epinephrine release. They may not be entirely benign, however, for in rare instances they can lead to acute renal failure due to acute tubular necrosis and occlusion of renal tubules by plugs of hemaceous material.

Renal function was measured in 56 runners before and after a 54-mile race. Urinary abnormalities appeared in 28. One of the runners had a decrease in creatine clearance when rechecked 3 weeks after the race, but a 5-month evaluation revealed normal renal function.

Unaccustomed strenuous exercise may induce renal damage due to a variety of mechanisms ranging from rhabdomyolysis, acidosis and hemolysis to temperature elevations, transient reductions in renal plasma flow and glomerular filtration rates, and reduction of urine volume. Koffler et al.[10] reported acute renal failure associated with nontraumatic rhabdomyolysis and myoglobinuria in 21 patients. In 18 of the 21, the illness followed overdoses of alcohol, heroin or other drugs, rather than athletic participation. Myoglobinuria differs from hemoglobinuria in that the urine shows few red blood cells and the serum is not pink, as it is in hemolytic hemoglobinuria. Muscle aching and weakness, along with serum protein elevations, provide additional clinical clues. Electrophoresis on starch gel or cellulose acetate, or absorption spectrophotometry and immunochemical techniques are other diagnostic methods.

Renal contusion is an occasional problem in contact sports, as evidenced by the following example:

A 32-year-old Atlanta Braves outfielder crashed into the left-field wall while chasing a fly ball. He was temporarily stunned but remained in the game. The following day he noticed that his urine was darker than usual, and when this persisted he notified the team trainer.

A urinalysis confirmed the presence of blood. The hemoglobin and blood urea nitrogen levels were normal. An intravenous pyelogram was likewise normal.

The player's activity was restricted for 3 days; he then returned to play as a pinch hitter. His urinalysis was normal within the 3-day period, and he returned to full activity after a week.

Polednak[11] studied mortality rates from renal disease of former college athletes, surveying 8,393 men who attended Harvard between 1880 and 1912. A comparison of athletes and nonathletes indicated no increased incidence of renal deaths in the former.

Venereal Disease

Venereal disease is not uncommon in athletes, especially in college and professional players.

The incubation period for syphilis is 2–6 weeks. The classic chancre is painless and accompanied by regional, painless adenopathy. Dark-field microscopy is the most reliable diagnostic tool. The VDRL may be positive within 4 weeks of exposure (and within 1 week after appearance of the lesion) but may remain negative in up to 28% of cases. The FTA-ABS test may miss 9%. The drug choice is benzathine penicillin, 2.4 million units intramuscularly. For persons allergic to penicillin, erythromycin may be given for 10 days.

Gonorrhea has a short incubation period of only 2–5 days and usually begins with the abrupt onset of dysuria and a purulent urethral discharge. A gram stain of the discharge shows intracellular diplococci. Treatment consists first of 1 gm of probenecid to enhance the serum level of the antibiotic of choice: 4.8 million units of aqueous procaine penicillin G intramuscularly, 3.5 gm of ampicillin, or 3 gm of Amoxicillin orally. Athletes allergic to penicillin can take 2 gm spectimomycin hydrochloride intramuscularly or oral tetracycline orally (1.5 gm initially, then 0.5 gm 4 times daily for 4 days).

Nongonococcal ("nonspecific") urethritis is common. It has been traced to two microorganisms (chlamydia and T-strain mycoplasmas), has an incubation period of 10–14 days and presents with a more gradual onset of milder symptoms than does gonorrhea. The patient and his sexual partner should be treated with 1.5 gm of tetracycline initially, followed by 0.5 gm every 6 hours for 1 week.

ENDOCRINE-METABOLIC DISORDERS

Diabetes Mellitus

Diabetes is a complex disorder, too vast to be effectively covered in a book of this nature. Standard medical texts (e.g., Beeson and McDermott's *Textbook of Medicine*) and monographs by the American Diabetes Association are highly recommended.

The athlete with diabetes should do the following:
1. Reduce body fat to less than 12% of total body weight;
2. Keep accurate records of sugar and acetone content of urine voided before meals and at bedtime;
3. Learn to recognize the early signs of insulin reactions, such as tremulousness, weakness and sweating;
4. Adhere to a strict diet, avoiding junk foods and excessive alcohol; and
5. Maintain regular endurance exercise habits.

The insulin dose should be reduced when prolonged endurance exercise is anticipated. Those taking NPH insulin should watch for hypoglycemic reactions during late-afternoon practice sessions, which occur at the peak of the drug's activity. All patients should switch to U-100 insulin to avoid possible errors in dosage administration.

Heat Stress

Heat stress[12-15] may present as one of 4 syndromes:
1. Heat cramps (probably a symptom of salt loss or of electrolyte shifts);
2. Heat fatigue (muscles don't function as efficiently as usual);
3. Heat exhaustion (weakness, sweating, dizziness, but no significant rise in temperature); or
4. Heat stroke (body temperature can rise to 105 F or higher).

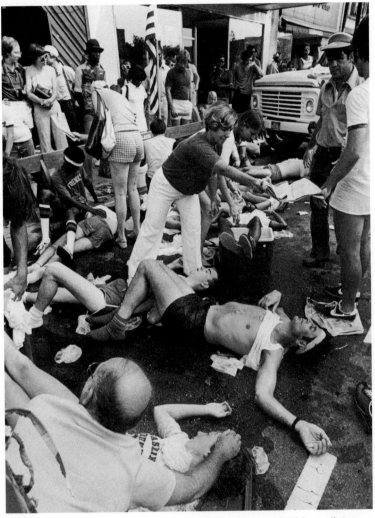

Fig 4–1.—Victims of heat exhaustion after a 10,000-m distance race in 88 F weather.

As both participants in, and postrace physicians for, the 10,000-m road race in Atlanta on July 4, we were impressed with the magnitude of heat-related illness (Fig 4–1). Approximately 60 of the nearly 6,000 finishers were taken by ambulance to a nearby hospital. Several of the subjects were critically ill; fortunately, there were no deaths. Most of the afflicted were average runners who pushed beyond their capabilities, perhaps trying too hard to win a coveted T-shirt (given to those who finished in less than 55 minutes) in 88 F weather.

In heat stroke, numerous body systems are involved. Central nervous system symptoms may indicate edema of brain tissue and petechial hemorrhages. Cardiac output is high, due to the increased demands on the circulatory system and the reduction in vascular resistance. Direct thermal injury to vascular endothelium can trigger consumption coagulopathy. Serum enzyme and bilirubin level may be increased, and centrolobular necrosis with cholestasis has infrequently been observed in fatal cases. Renal manifestations may include acute tubular necrosis (seen in 10–35% of cases), which may be due to direct thermal injury, to myoglobinuria and to a diminution of renal blood flow. Up to 15–20 gm of salt and approximately 500 mg of potassium can be lost in a day.

Hypokalemia is seen in 50% of patients with acute heat stroke. This may be due partly to hyperventilation with secondary alkalosis, which drives the potassium into the cell, although up to 100 mEq or more of potassium can be lost in sweat per day.

The treatment of heat stroke includes vigorous massage, ice baths and phenothiazines (to reduce shivering). Fluid replacement should begin with administration of Ringer's lactate; the average fluid need in the first 4 hours is 1,400 ml. Mannitol may be used to increase renal blood flow and promote diuresis. Oxygen should be given if the pO_2 is below 65 mm Hg. If congestive heart failure is present, with rales in the lungs and a typical chest x-ray appearance, diuretics and digitalis can be used. Serum electrolytes must be watched closely. In severe heart failure or hypotension, a Swan-Ganz catheter should be used to monitor the left ventricular (LV) filling pressure. If hypotension is accompanied by a low filling pressure, fluid should be administered until the pulmonary capillary wedge pressure (or LV filling pressure) is 16–18 mm Hg. If hypotension persists despite an adequate filling pressure, dopamine is the drug of choice. Infrequently, disseminated intravascular coagulation will necessitate therapy with heparin (1 in 41 instances in O'Donnell's report).[15]

The most important therapeutic measure pertaining to heat stroke is prevention. Greater emphasis on fluid replacement before, during and after athletic participation has reduced the incidence of this disorder. The fluid should be cold, as cold solutions are emptied from the stomach faster than warm ones. It should contain less than 2.5 gm of glucose per 100 ml of water, for higher concentrations increase the osmolality and reduce the rate of gastric emptying. The glucose is needed to avoid hypoglycemia in endurance events. Remember that, in the initial phase of such events, most of the metabolized carbohydrate comes from muscle glycogen and eventually from liver glycogen. When the liver output cannot keep up with the muscle needs, hypoglycemia can result unless glucose is provided from external sources. The glucose taken up across the intestinal wall is stored in the liver as glycogen. Unlike liver glycogen, some of which is restored after only one meal, muscle glycogen takes up to 48 hours to replace. Salt tablets are best avoided, for athletes are already hypernatremic (since sweat is hypotonic), and they may not drink adequate amounts of water with the tablets.

Distance races ranging from 6 to 26 miles are becoming commonplace, especially during the summer. We make the following recommendations to those participating in such events:

1. Do not enter the race as a lark. Remember the words of Alexander Pope: "Fools rush in where angels fear to tread."
2. Do not experiment with diets before the race. Some runners who have suffered heat exhaustion followed unsound nutritional practices such as going without solid food for several days or trying their own version of carbohydrate loading (see Chap. 9) for the first time.
3. In warm weather, drink a glass or two of fluid a half hour

before a 6+-mile race. Try the fluid during training runs so you are sure it is well-tolerated.

4. Do not run if you have a flulike illness with fever and muscle aches. Remember the experimental studies where myocarditis was produced in animals by exposing them to a virus and then exercising them.

5. Race to your own drummer, to paraphrase Thoreau. Forget about trying to beat your neighbor. Set a realistic goal. Do not start out too fast on courses that begin with a mile or so downhill.

We advise canceling races longer than 10 miles when the wet bulb–globe temperature exceeds 82.4 F (28 C), a policy advocated by the American College of Sports Medicine. To calculate the wet bulb–globe temperature (WB-GT), the following formula is used:

$$WB\text{-}GT = 0.7 \text{ (wet bulb temp.)} + 0.2 \text{ (globe temp.)} \\ + 0.1 \text{ (dry bulb temp.).}$$

Fluid stations should be set up at 2-mile intervals, even in races of only 6 miles, when such events are held in warm, humid weather. Efforts should be made to start these races in the early morning (8:00 A.M.) or late afternoon (4:00 P.M.). The emphasis should be on participation, and T-shirts and related memorabilia should be given to all who finish the event, regardless of time.

Weight Control

Body-composition analysis, using the skinfold-caliper technique or hydrostatic weighing, is useful in determining an athlete's ideal body weight. Because there is no advantage to having more than 14% of total body weight as fat, we advise athletes to keep below this level. Nutritional counseling is recommended for those who are unable to regulate caloric intake on their own. "Gimmick" diets are to be avoided, and athletes should be educated about the merits of a combined approach—increased caloric expenditure plus decreased caloric intake.

Those wishing to gain muscle mass should likewise be educated as to how this can only be accomplished by increasing muscle work, with a corresponding increase in food intake. They should be told that muscle protein cannot be increased by eating foods high in protein, contrary to popular belief. The diet should contain foods other than those with saturated animal fats and refined carbohydrates.

Crash weight-gain and weight-loss programs, such as the ones followed by many wrestling teams, are to be condemned, as should the use of anabolic steroids.

For several days before athletic competition the diet should be rich in nonrefined carbohydrates. Carbohydrate loading should be avoided because of potential hazards of muscle heaviness and stiffness (due to water deposition), possible muscle fiber destruction and perhaps even ECG changes with angina-like chest pain. The advice of Cooper and Fair seems prudent:

> The content of the pregame meal is not critical as long as it does not make the athlete sick, uncomfortable, irritate his gastrointestinal tract, markedly delay the emptying time of his stomach. Far more important is the combination of diet and exercise during the week preceding competition.[16]

HEMATOLOGY

Sickle Cell Trait[17]

Sickle cell trait is found in up to 10% of the black population. It is important to screen all black athletes for this condition, as several deaths have been reported in afflicted persons who have engaged in vigorous exercise. It is advisable to avoid hypoxic conditions (e.g., prolonged exercise at high altitude), which may produce sickling. Lactic acidosis may aggravate the condition.

Athletes with sickle cell trait should be observed for any signs of exertional rhabdomyolysis, in which hydration, prompt correction of acidosis and oxygenation are indicated.

"Sports" Anemia

The mild anemia seen occasionally in athletes has been attributed to various causes. It could indicate subclinical hemolysis of red blood cells circulating through the feet, caused by trauma to the feet as they strike hard pavement. Hemosiderin might be shed in the urine in such instances. The anemia might also be due to a loss of iron in sweat, which contains 0.4 mg iron per liter; therefore, a vigorous endurance workout with a 10-L sweat loss could result in a 4-mg loss of iron. Additional studies may be helpful in expanding knowledge of this condition.

NEUROPSYCHIATRIC PROBLEMS

Headaches

Migraine-like syndromes are variable during periods of exercise. Some athletes with this condition think that exercise is beneficial; others find that it aggravates the headache. Regular eating habits and ample sleep are important. Sublingual ergotamine tartrate (Ergomar) may be helpful if taken at the initial onset of discomfort. A second tablet may be taken 30 minutes later if pain persists. Propranolol may also be tried.

Seizures

Athletes with well-controlled seizure disorders (epilepsy) may participate in sports. Livingston et al.,[18] describing several hundred such individuals over a 36-year period, did not "know of a single instance of recurrence of epileptic seizures related to head injury in any of these athletes." Team physicians should include intravenous phenobarbital and diazepam (Valium) in their emergency drug kits for treatment of these disorders.

Head Injuries and Concussions[19–21]

Schneider[21] classifies cerebral concussions as follows:
First degree.—There is no loss of consciousness, but the athlete may be slightly confused. He may also experience dizziness and ringing in the ears (thus the sports cliché, "getting your bell rung").
Second degree.—The athlete loses consciousness but recovers within 5 minutes. He may be slightly unsteady and confused upon regaining consciousness.
Third degree.—The player is unconscious for more than 5 minutes. He is unsteady and confused after regaining consciousness and may complain of severe dizziness and ringing of the ears.

Athletes who complain of severe neck pain after regaining consciousness should be assumed to have a cervical spine injury until proved otherwise. They should be transported to a medical facility for x-rays and a neurological examination on a rigid spine board, with the head and neck stabilized to prevent movement. If the individual is wearing a helmet, it should not be removed.

Players with third-degree concussion should be evaluated in a medical facility and should not return to the game in which they were injured. The management of those with lesser degrees of concussion must be individualized. As a general rule, the high-school athlete should be held out of the remainder of the game if he has lost consciousness for several minutes. Key college and professional players are sometimes returned to action, provided a sideline neurological assessment is normal and they do not have a persistent headache.

Emotional Disorders

Psychiatric problems in athletes should be handled by a professional counselor. Discretion should be used at the professional level to prevent information "leaks" to the mass media. Lesser emotional problems can usually be handled by the team physician, who is often close to the players and has earned their trust and confidence.

The team doctor should be alert for any signs of drug abuse and should not go along in any way with such practices as the use of "diet pills" for pregame "uppers." Professional athletes should be discouraged from excessive postgame beer drinking, which can sometimes lead to chronic alcoholism, as in the case of former Dodger pitcher Don Newcombe (who now counsels others with this problem).

MISCELLANEOUS PROBLEMS

Choking and Resuscitation

The trainer and all members of the coaching staff should be trained in cardiopulmonary resuscitation (CPR), including the Heimlich maneuver[22] for choking victims. The former manager of the Atlanta Braves can be thankful that pitching coach

Herman Starrette knew this maneuver, for Starrette success-fully applied it when the manager was choking on a piece of meat.

Following collisions in such noncontact sports as baseball and basketball, the unconscious player may "swallow his tongue." This is caused by relaxation of the oropharyngeal muscles, allowing the tongue to fall back in the throat and oc-clude the airway. This passage must be promptly opened by tilting the victim's head back while supporting the neck with the other hand. If this is not immediately successful, pull for-ward on the mandible (while tilting the head back) or use a choke-saver to pull the tongue forward. One must, of course, be extremely careful not to manipulate the cervical spine if any injury in this area is suspected.

Food Poisoning

When several members of a team suddenly develop gas-trointestinal signs and symptoms such as pain, vomiting and diarrhea, food poisoning should be suspected. Staphylococcus infections develop within 1–6 hours after eating and usually subside within 8 hours. Clostridium perfringens infections have an incubation period of 6–24 hours (usually 8–12 hr); the illness usually subsides within a day. Diarrhea is treated as outlined on page 52. Persistent emesis generally responds to intramuscular injection of prochlorperazine (Compazine), 10 mg every 6 hours if necessary. Clostridium botulinum infec-tions are fortunately rare but should be considered when se-vere gastrointestinal symptoms are followed or accompanied by such neurologic symptoms as visual blurring, difficulty in swallowing or speaking and progressive muscle weakness. Victims should be hospitalized and treated with antitoxin.

Menstrual Disorders[23]

Strenuous sports activity may cause various menstrual disor-ders. Scanty menstrual flow, and even prolonged amenorrhea, is not uncommon in female distance runners. In seasonal sports, such as rowing, the symptoms subside during the months of rest.

A thorough gynecologic history and physical examination

are indicated. If no other cause can be found, the athlete should be counseled to reduce the intensity of training and should be reassured that there is nothing to be concerned about.

Common Skin Problems

Athlete's Foot

Tinea pedis, also known as ringworm of the foot, commonly produces itching, fissure formation and inflammation with erythema. Fungal infections of the toenails may be a concomitant finding. The diagnosis can be confirmed by microscopic examinations of a KOH preparation from the involved area. The condition is common and usually responds to ointments or creams containing haloprogin (Halotex) or tolnaftate (Tinactin).

Groin Rashes

So-called jock itch is usually due to Tinea cruris (ringworm of the groin), although it may also be caused by monilia (a condition known as intertrigo). If the lesion is dry, does not involve the scrotum and has a well-demarcated border, tinea is likely. It responds to heloprogin or tolnaftate. If the lesion is moist, involves the scrotum and has satellite pustules or an indistinct border, monilia is likely. This yeast can be treated with Mycostatin powder or cream or with clotrimazole (Lotrimin) cream.

REFERENCES

1. Ferguson, A., Addington, W. W., and Gaensler, E. A.: Dyspnea and bronchospasm from inappropriate postexercise hyperventilation, Ann. Intern. Med. 71:1063, 1969.
2. Katz, R. M.: Asthmatics don't have to sit out sports, Phys. Sports Med. 4:45, 1976.
3. Shephard, R. J.: Exercise-induced bronchospasm—a review, Med. Sci. Sports 9:1, 1977.
4. Bierman, C. W., Pierson, W. E., and Shapiro, G. G.: Exercise-induced asthma, J.A.M.A. 234:295, 1975.
5. Wilson, R.: Acute high-altitude illness in mountaineers and problems of rescue, Ann. Intern. Med. 78:421, 1973.
6. Kleiner, J. P., and Nelson, W. P.: High-altitude pulmonary edema: a rare disease? J.A.M.A. 234:491, 1975.

7. Krissoff, W. B., and Eiseman, B.: The hazards of exercising at altitude, Phys. Sports Med. 3:26, 1975.

8. Van Liere, E. J.: Postrace diarrhea, J.A.M.A. 236:604, 1976.

9. Gardner, K. D., Jr.: Athletic nephritis: pseudo and real, Ann. Intern. Med. 75:966, 1971.

10. Koffler, A., Friedler, R. M., and Massry, S. G.: Acute renal failure due to nontraumatic rhabdomyolysis, Ann. Intern. Med. 85:23, 1976.

11. Polednak, A. P.: Mortality from renal diseases among former college athletes, Ann. Intern. Med. 77:919, 1972.

12. Knochel, J. P.: Dog days and siriasis: how to kill a football player, J.A.M.A. 233:513, 1975.

13. Clowes, G. H. A., Jr., and O'Donnell, T. F., Jr.: Heat stroke, N. Engl. J. Med. 291:564, 1974.

14. Balancing heat stress, fluids, and electrolytes, Phys. Sports Med. 3:43, 1975.

15. O'Donnell, T. F., Jr.: Acute heat stroke, J.A.M.A. 234:824, 1975.

16. Cooper, D. L., and Fair, J.: Pregame meal: to eat or not to eat— and what? Phys. Sports Med. 4:37, 1976.

17. Panel discussion: Should sickle cell trait bar sports participation? Phys. Sports Med. 4:58, 1976.

18. Livingston, S., and Berman, W.: Participation of epileptic patients in sports, J.A.M.A. 224:236, 1973.

19. Forg, J. S., and Quedensfeld, T. C.: When the athlete's life is threatened, Phys. Sports Med. 3:54, 1975.

20. Ryan, A. J.: On-field diagnosis of head injuries, Phys. Sports Med. 4:82, 1976.

21. Schneider, R.: *Head and Neck Injuries in Football* (Baltimore: Williams & Wilkins Co., 1973).

22. Heimlich, H. J.: A life-saving maneuver to prevent food-choking, J.A.M.A. 234:398, 1975.

23. Erdelyi, G. J.: Effects of exercise on the menstrual cycle, Phys. Sports Med. 4:79, 1976.

5 / Cardiovascular Problems and Physical Activity

The athlete is subject to the same cardiovascular diseases as the average person. To complicate matters, the physically active individual may have some physiological variations from normal that can be misconstrued as indicative of disease by the uninitiated. A thorough data base (including the medical history, physical examination and noninvasive laboratory studies), together with experience in the normal variants of the athlete's heart, generally clarifies the issue. Infrequently, one must rely upon an invasive study, such as cardiac catheterization, for the final answer.

In this chapter we will review the methods and techniques of obtaining a good cardiac data base and the utilization of the problem-oriented method to illustrate the varieties of cardiac disease and nondisease that one might encounter in the athlete.

THE CARDIOVASCULAR DATA BASE

The athlete should be asked about any past diseases that might have involved the heart, such as rheumatic fever and serious viral illnesses. He or she should be specifically questioned regarding symptoms referable to the heart or lungs, such as shortness of breath, palpitations, productive cough, syncope or near-syncope, ankle edema, paroxysmal nocturnal dyspnea and chest pain. The physician should not be content just to inquire about "pain" but should ask about any sensations in the chest such as "fullness," "tightness" and the like. Individuals may deny having any exertional chest pain but will admit to a viselike gripping beneath the sternum when jogging or engaging in other vigorous activities.

The physical examination of the cardiovascular system should be performed in a quiet room, rather than in a noisy gymnasium. The blood pressure should be checked in both arms, for it may vary in supravalvular aortic stenosis and in coarctation of the aorta. If the arm pressure is elevated, the pressure must be measured in the legs in search for coarctation. The pulse should be studied for at least a minute, looking for any irregularities of the cardiac rate or rhythm. All major pulse sites (carotid, radial, aorta, femoral, popliteal, dorsalis

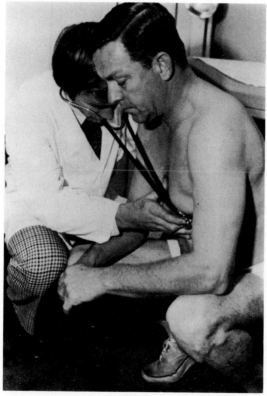

Fig 5–1. — Examination of the heart with patient in squatting position.

pedis, posterior tibial) should be graded on a 0–4 scale, with 3 being normal. The pupils should be dilated to permit an adequate inspection of the optic fundi.

The neck is examined for carotid bruits, venous hums, neck vein distention and thyroid enlargement. The chest is percussed and auscultated, for bruits or murmurs transmitting to the back and for any signs of bronchoconstriction.

The cardiac area is inspected and palpated to localize the point of maximal impulse. The apex impulse should also be palpated with the subject in the left lateral position. Auscultation of the heart is done in a systematic way, listening in the aortic, pulmonic, tricuspid and mitral areas to the first and second heart sounds in systole and diastole, noting any clicks, gallops or murmurs. The standard auscultation is done with the subject in the supine, sitting and left lateral positions. In the latter position, the examiner should use the bell, after first exercising the subject, to search for the low-frequency rumble of mitral stenosis. The physician should also listen to the heart with the subject in the standing and the squatting positions (Fig 5–1), which may produce significant variations in the click-murmur syndrome and in idiopathic hypertrophic subaortic stenosis (IHSS).

If a systolic murmur is detected, it should be graded on a 1–6 scale. Innocent (or physiologic "flow" murmurs) are seldom grade 3 or more in intensity. One should also observe the effects of the following maneuvers on the murmur: respiration, Valsalva, hand grip, exercise (sit-ups or running in place) and position of maximum and minimum intensity.

Carefully palpate the abdomen, feeling for enlargement of the liver or spleen and excessive lateral expansion of the aorta. It is also important to auscultate in all 4 abdominal quadrants, the flanks and the low-back regions for vascular bruits.

The extremities are viewed for signs of clubbing, cyanosis and edema.

Routine laboratory studies include a blood count and urinalysis. It would be good to obtain a blood cholesterol level, particularly if there is a family history of coronary disease before age 60. A blood sugar test is advised if there is a family history of diabetes.

An electrocardiogram is advisable, but not essential, for the high-school or college athlete. It should be obtained if the cardiac examination reveals any abnormalities. An exercise stress test, using the treadmill or bicycle, can be done in selected instances to assess the effect of exercise on the rhythm and the blood pressure.

The echocardiogram provides an invaluable, new, noninvasive way to screen for congenital, valvular, pericardial and myocardial disease whenever the physical examination indi-

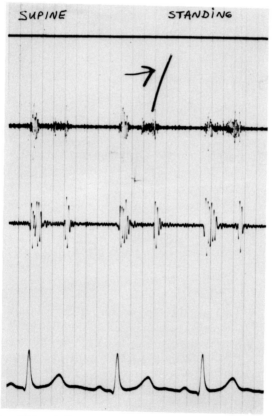

Fig 5–2. — Midsystolic click, followed by late systolic murmur (Barlow's syndrome or mitral valve prolapse) in a former college halfback.

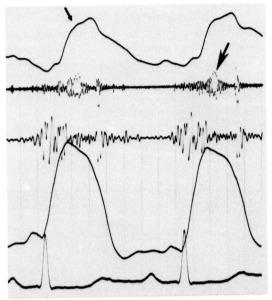

Fig 5–3. — Delayed carotid upstroke *(small arrow)* and systolic ejection murmur *(large arrow)* in a young athlete with aortic stenosis.

cates a likelihood of this. Graphic recordings (phono- and apexcardiograms, carotid and jugular pulse tracings) may occasionally be helpful, particularly in the click-murmur syndrome (Fig 5–2), aortic stenosis (Fig 5–3) and IHSS.

CARDIAC NONDISEASE IN ATHLETES

Clarence DeMar, the legendary Boston Marathoner, was one of the first patients with cardiac "nondisease." A systolic heart murmur was detected in Mr. DeMar after he had completed his first marathon; it was 8 years before he would again compete in this event. A diastolic heart sound was also recorded in DeMar and was most likely a ventricular filling sound (or S_3 gallop), which is not unusual in a young, thin-chested, normal distance runner.

The normal athlete may have a sinus bradycardia. The left ventricular impulse may be forceful. An atrial contraction sound (or S_4 gallop) is often heard, and vascular bruits that indicate the increase in stroke volume may also be detected. These physical findings should not be misinterpreted as symptoms of a disease state.

The chest x-ray may show cardiac enlargement in the normal athlete, a reflection of left ventricular hypertrophy. The electrocardiogram is frequently abnormal, particularly in endurance athletes and in black athletes. One of the participants in the recent international marathon race for women stated that the examining physician was concerned about her prerace electrocardiogram because it was not abnormal! Left ventricular hypertrophy is a common ECG finding. Variations in the repolarization pattern may be misinterpreted as pericarditis or myocardial injury. Right bundle-branch block, 2d-degree A-V block of the Wenckebach type, a wandering atrial pacemaker, supraventricular and ventricular premature beats, and left axis deviation have all been recorded in otherwise normal athletes.

Echocardiography in normal athletes may reveal increased left and right ventricular end-diastolic dimensions and increases in left ventricular wall thickness. This will differ from the heart hypertrophied from disease in that the ejection fractions and velocity of circumferential fiber shortening of the left ventricle will be normal (or even supranormal). The septal-left ventricular posterior wall thickness ratios may exceed the upper normal limit of 1.3. This might be a normal variant in athletes, but one should search for other clues (such as a systolic heart murmur that is markedly intensified upon Valsalva's maneuver or when standing, and systolic anterior movement of the anterior leaflet of the mitral valve on echo) to suggest IHSS. The latter contraindicates vigorous exercise, as it has produced effort-related sudden deaths, including a recent instance involving a college basketball player.

CARDIAC DISEASE

The spectrum of cardiovascular problems encountered in the physically active individual can best be considered under the following categorization, using several examples from the private practice of one of the authors (JDC).

Congenital Heart Disease

A 26-year-old man with a known ventricular septal defect was referred for an exercise prescription. Examination showed a normal-sized heart, and there was no suggestion of pulmonary hypertension. The ECG and chest x-ray were normal. A previous cardiac catheterization indicated a left-to-right shunt of 1.4 to 1. The man was cleared for vigorous physical activity. If the heart had been enlarged or if the flow ratio had been greater than 1.75 to 1, strenuous exercise would have been proscribed and surgical closure strongly considered. A similar approach can be taken in the patient with an atrial septal defect, although, generally, these patients more often come to surgery than do those with ventricular septal defects. Spontaneous closure of the atrial defects occurs less frequently than closure of ventricular septal defects.

Surgical closure is usually recommended when a patent ductus arteriosus is discovered, even when the lesion is small, for the risk of endocarditis is probably higher than the ex-

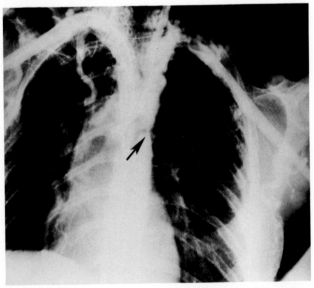

Fig 5–4. — Coarctation of the aorta in a 20-year-old female college basketball player.

tremely low risk of surgical repair. Physical activity need not be restricted unless pulmonary hypertension is present.

Coarctation of the aorta is possible in a young athlete with hypertension, especially if a systolic ejection murmur is heard in the mid-back area. A 20-year-old woman complained of excessive fatigue when playing basketball. Her school physical had revealed mild hypertension. Careful examination showed diminished femoral pulses and leg blood pressures that were less than the arm pressure. Subsequent cardiac catheterization confirmed the clinical diagnosis of coarctation (Fig 5–4), and the patient underwent surgical repair. In the absence of severe hypertension on follow-up, she would be cleared for all recreational activity.

Patients with mild aortic or pulmonic stenosis (i.e., no ventricular hypertrophy on chest x-ray or ECG, an outflow gradient of < 40 mm Hg) may be athletically inclined and need not be restricted. Close clinical follow-up is advised, however, for both lesions may be progressive.

Considerable recent attention has been given to Barlow's syndrome, which may be detected in the athlete. A 30-year-old former college football and baseball player had been told of a heart murmur on several occasions but had never been given a precise assessment of it. Auscultation revealed a mid-systolic click, followed by a late systolic murmur at the apex. The murmur intensified with standing. The heart was not enlarged and the resting and exercise-stress rhythm remained stable. He was okayed for a home jogging program.

Rare congenital conditions, such as anomalous coronary arteries and coronary arteriovenous fistulas, have been implicated in myocardial infarctions and sudden death in young athletes.

Coronary Atherosclerotic Heart Disease

The tragic sudden death of a professional football player on national television, a death attributed to extensive coronary disease, emphasizes that the athlete is not immune to this disease. This is not surprising in view of autopsy studies on young soldiers and victims of auto accidents.

The preseason medical evaluation should include a thorough family history, with the examiner looking for instances of premature coronary events (i.e., infarction, angina, sudden death) prior to age 55–60 in close relatives. In the event of the latter, the athlete's skin should be scrutinized for lipid deposits, and serum cholesterol and triglyceride levels should be obtained.

Athletes who complain of exertional chest pain that subsides with rest should be studied with exercise stress testing. Repeated questioning, a trial of nitroglycerin and exercise under medical supervision may be in order. Infrequently, one must rely on coronary arteriography.

Chest pain may occur in IHSS; sometimes the ECG may resemble that of coronary disease. Similarly, chest pain may occur during or after the tachycardia phase of the Wolff-Parkinson-White syndrome, and the δ wave on the ECG may simulate the Q wave of transmural infarction to the casual reader.

Cor Pulmonale

Cor pulmonale has not been a problem in my experience. The person with underlying lung disease severe enough to produce secondary heart dysfunction will not tolerate strenuous physical exertion.

Hypertension and Vascular Disease

The athlete with persistent hypertension should be evaluated for curable causes, such as coarctation of the aorta, renal disease and adrenal disorders. If the blood pressure is consistently above 160/100 mm Hg, the response to exercise should be ascertained on the treadmill. If the systolic pressure rises above 220 mm Hg, or the diastolic pressure above 110 mm Hg, vigorous physical activity (e.g., track, swimming, football) is curtailed. Sustained hypertension should be treated with salt restriction and, if there is excess body fat, a low-calorie diet. If the blood pressure continues to be higher than 160/95 mm Hg, a diuretic is added, followed by more potent agents if necessary. The step-care approach to the pharmacologic therapy of hypertension, as described by the American Heart Association, is a logical way to proceed.

Vascular problems are uncommon in athletes. Thrombophlebitis may develop after sports-related trauma or in an athlete temporarily immobilized after orthopedic surgery. Thrombophlebitis of the deep veins of the leg may lead to pulmonary embolism.

Arterial disorders are even less common in the athlete. One type to watch for, particularly in basketball players, is a dissecting aneurysm of the thoracic aorta. A college basketball star with unrecognized Marfan's syndrome had this as a terminal event during a half-court pickup scrimmage. It may occur in other types of athletes. I am currently following a mesomorphic former college baseball player who developed chest pain and a murmur of aortic regurgitation and eventually had surgical repair of a thoracic aortic aneurysm.

Rheumatic Fever

Acute rheumatic fever is no longer as common in youngsters as in years past. The practice of culturing sore throats and treating streptococcal infection with intramuscular benzathine penicillin or a 10-day oral penicillin regimen has been helpful in reducing the prevalence of the rheumatic sequelae.

Nonetheless, it is not rare to discover murmurs on preseason physical examinations that may be residua of subclinical rheumatic fever years ago (or rheumatic fever that masqueraded as a nonspecific viral illness). The mitral valve is usually involved in rheumatic carditis, and the aortic valve may be concomitantly diseased. It is unusual to have isolated aortic valve disease due to rheumatic carditis.

The athlete with mitral regurgitation need not be limited if the heart size on ECG and chest x-ray are normal, there are no symptoms, and a maximum treadmill stress test is normal. An example is a 13-year-old boy with a history of rheumatic carditis at age 6, and a murmur of mitral regurgitation since that time. His cardiac size is normal on chest x-ray and on ECG, and his exercise stress test is also normal. Consequently, he is not restricted in his sports activities. Vigorous sports are not recommended when the heart has begun to enlarge; but hiking, golf, tennis doubles and other less strenuous activities may be enjoyed. Mitral stenosis is a contraindication to vigorous sports, even when the heart is of normal size. Aortic stenosis is managed as in the congenital variety. Aortic regurgitation can be managed like mitral regurgitation.

Rhythm Problems

Supraventricular premature beats may result in palpitations, anxiety, chest sensations and hyperventilation. A college halfback became concerned about irregular heart beats and subsequently noted chest discomfort. His cardiac examination was normal, as was a resting ECG and chest x-ray. On treadmill stress testing his symptoms were reproduced, coinciding with occasional supraventricular premature beats. He was simply reassurred and advised to enhance his level of physical fitness, which was only in the "average" category for his age group, as measured by oxygen-uptake analysis. He had a fine senior year with no further difficulties.

Ventricular premature beats (VPBs) have been recorded in high-school track stars and football players, in addition to

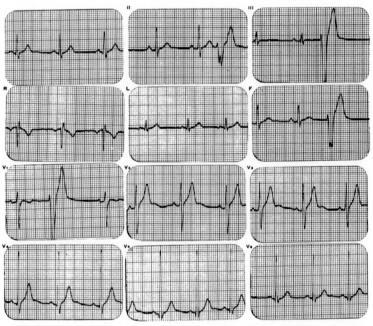

Fig 5–5. — Ventricular premature beats in resting ECG of an amateur runner.

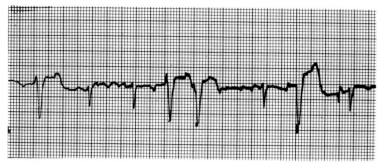

Fig 5–6. — Marked ventricular irritability in a veteran Boston Marathon runner who collapsed while running.

amateur runners (Fig 5–5). Generally, these require no special treatment other than reassurance if the cardiac evaluation is otherwise normal and if the extrasystoles are suppressed with exercise testing. If the VPBs are accentuated with exercise, if they are multifocal or near the vulnerable period of the ECG, or if they occur in runs of 2 or more, vigorous exercise should be curtailed and close medical follow-up instituted. Life-threatening problems can arise if this is not done, as evidenced by a veteran Boston Marathoner who had to be resuscitated on 2 occasions while running because of ventricular tachycardia (Fig 5–6).

Paroxysmal atrial tachyarrhythmias are sometimes a problem to the athlete. If they occur more frequently than once every 6 months or so, digitalis may help to prevent them.

Pericardial Disease

Congenital defects of the pericardium may mimic more serious cardiac diseases on ECG and chest x-ray; they usually need not limit physical activity.

Acquired pericarditis may be due to a variety of illnesses but is most often viral or idiopathic. A precise diagnosis is important, for residual ECG changes may mimic coronary disease and lead to unnecessary limitations.

A former college athlete developed chest pain after knee surgery. Pericarditis was diagnosed from the ECG (Fig 5–7),

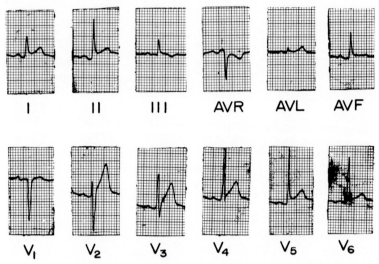

Fig 5—7. — Acute pericarditis in a former college athlete.

and serial ECGs (Fig 5–8) supported this diagnosis. As soon as the ECG returned to normal and his knee permitted, he was cleared for all athletic activities.

Endomyocardial Disease

Bacterial endocarditis is a potential threat to any athlete with an organic heart murmur who does not follow endocarditis prophylaxis for dental work or any operative procedures.

Myocardial disease may be primary or secondary. The former, which includes IHSS, precludes vigorous exercise. In fact, some physicians have suggested strict, prolonged bed rest as the therapy of choice for certain types (although this is not usually feasible).

The myocardium may be involved in many types of disorders, including vasculitides, infection, toxins, autoimmune and allergic diseases, metabolic disorders and neoplasms. These are rare diseases, but occasionally can involve the athlete, as evidenced by the local college football lineman who succumbed to leptospirosis of the heart.

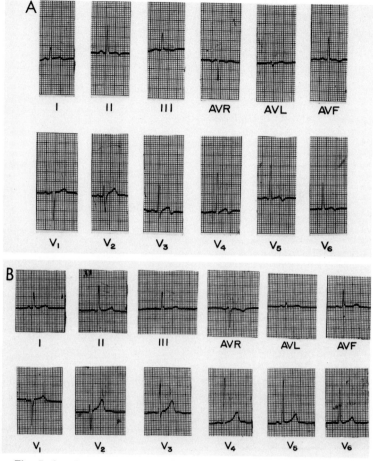

Fig 5–8.—A and **B,** serial ECGs in subject described in Figure 5–7.

SUMMARY

The techniques of collecting a cardiovascular data base for an athlete have been discussed, together with features of the normal athlete's heart that may mimic cardiac disease. A spectrum of organic heart disease in athletes has been presented.

The statement by the Ad Hoc Committee on Habilitation of the Young Cardiac[1] is a useful guide for the team physician in deciding which sports can be permitted and which must be proscribed.

REFERENCE

1. Council on cardiovascular diseases in the young, American Heart Association: Activity guidelines for young patients with heart disease. Phys Sports Med. 4:47, 1976.

6 / Orthopedic Evaluation of the Athlete in the Office

Examination of the injured athlete in the office can be done in a relaxed, orderly manner without pressure from coaches, the crowd and other players. Many problems seen in the office are similar to those seen in the arena. Fractures, dislocations, third-degree sprains and tendon ruptures may be seen some time after the onset of the acute problem because there was no medical attention at the time of injury. Or the athlete may have thought his injury a minor one, not mentioning it until the problem failed to clear within 24–48 hours.

Problems that are more likely to occur in the arena will be discussed in Chapter 7. The majority of the problems discussed in the following paragraphs are produced by athletic endeavors that involve repetitive movements, such as running, rowing, cycling, tennis or swimming. The symptoms are often vague, and the physical findings may not be dramatic. Nevertheless, close attention must be paid to the athlete's complaint, a thorough examination performed and an accurate diagnosis made. Only then will treatment be effective, allowing the patient to resume activity that may be a very important facet in his life.

EXERCISE HISTORY

As in any other field of medicine, the patient's history is very important. Many diagnoses come from the history alone. The history obtained in the office will be more detailed than that in the arena. With the increased popularity of repetitive physical fitness activities, many areas of the history and physical examination that were previously considered insignificant may become meaningful.

The exact nature of the patient's complaint must be determined. This is often obtained not by asking, "What is wrong with you?" but, "What have you noticed that is different?" Once the exact area of the problem has been identified, step-by-step questioning about the development of the symptoms should be undertaken. Questioning should determine whether a single episode started the problem or whether the problem gradually developed over a period of time. Inquiries must be made about what exacerbates the symptoms and what makes them abate. Learning whether there has been any change in athletic equipment or whether old equipment has been repaired is important. It is also necessary to know if there has been any change in the exercise patterns or in the exercise environment. Finally, it is necessary to ask about the results of any prior treatment, either professional or self-administered. Often many remedies have already been tried and discarded with partial or no success.

Following a detailed history of the present complaint, some general information should be obtained. Has the patient had previous problems with his bones or joints in other areas? Does the patient know of any discrepancy in leg lengths or size of the extremities? Does he know of any growth disturbances or childhood problems? What are the patient's present occupation and other recreational interests? Last, it is important to know if the patient has any serious illnesses, such as heart or lung disease, or systemic problems, such as diabetes or gout. It is also important to know if the athlete is taking any medication.

In summary, an athlete will most frequently consult a physician for 3 complaints: pain, a loss of physical competence indicating a decrease in function, or an alteration in physical appearance, such as malalignment of an extremity, swelling or alteration in gait.

PHYSICAL EXAMINATION

Physical examination of the athlete should be approached in a systematic way, which includes inspection, palpation, auscultation and special testing, which, in the case of the musculoskeletal system, includes assessment of joint motion and neurologic function.

The affected area should be examined without clothing, and if that area is an extremity, the opposite extremity should also be examined. The general demeanor of the athlete, his body habitus and the way he carries himself should be observed. The skin should be checked for abnormal color and texture, for any surgical scars and for any draining areas, atrophy or hypertrophy. The limbs should be measured for length discrepancy. Circumferential measurements of the extremities at different levels determine equality of muscle mass. Fortunately, the opposite unaffected limb is available to make comparison easy. Watching the patient move will provide information about pain. For example, if the patient walks with a limp due to pain, the stride length on the hurting side will be shortened (antalgic gait).

Palpation will help in several areas. Skin temperature can be noted by carefully comparing one side of the body to the other. Increase in skin temperature usually indicates a vascular response, the most common cause of which is inflammation. The bony prominences should be palpated to find any tender areas, thickness, malalignment or swelling. If there is swelling, is it due to thickness of the tissues in the region of tenderness? Is the swelling fluid within the joint? Is the swelling generalized pitting edema? If the swelling is intra-articular, it is generally reactive fluid for the protection of the joint. If the joint swelling has been present for a long time, obtaining a sample of the fluid for gross and microscopic examination may be helpful.

Local tenderness is very important and must be clearly identified. If possible, the exact anatomical structure that is creating the tenderness should be determined. The physician can palpate along the courses of each of the anatomical structures about the joint to determine the exact area. If the joint is stressed by passive motion or by valgus or varus strain and the symptoms are reproduced, the problem is either in the joint capsule or in the ligaments. If active rather than passive motion reproduces symptoms, the injured structure is probably the musculotendinous unit. Unfortunately, because of the contiguity of structures it may be impossible to accurately delineate the offending anatomical structure.

Auscultation

Auscultation is not as important in the musculoskeletal examination as it is in other parts of the general physical examination. Crepitus, a grating sound, is important if it is present. Crepitus can be felt in the areas of fractures; it should alert the examiner to be gentle and curtail further physical examination until x-rays have been obtained. There could also be crepitus over the joints, particularly the knee. On flexion-extension of the knee joint, roughness underneath the patella may produce palpable, if not audible, crepitus. Swollen tendons moving over each other may produce a snapping type of crepitus. Although seldom used in this part of an examination, listening over a joint with a stethoscope may be of value in determining what is going on within that joint.

Special Tests

Measurements of extremities can be important, especially in the lower extremities, because the majority of exercise-related problems occur there. It has been taught that up to half an inch of leg-length discrepancy is within normal limits, but in many repetitive activities, such as jogging, a half inch may be important. There are several methods of measuring. The simplest is to observe the standing patient from behind to see if one iliac crest is higher than the other. A more precise measurement is made with the patient lying down. With the anterior superior iliac spine or the umbilicus as a proximal marking point, the medial malleolus can be used as the distal reference point and measurements taken.

Another frequently helpful measurement is the circumference of a limb. For example, the size of the forearm muscle mass can be ascertained by using the tip of the olecranon as a reference point. The circumference of the muscles can be measured 2 inches below the tip of the olecranon on each side and compared, giving a rough idea of muscle equality. Other reference points, such as the superior pole of the patella, can be used for the legs.

Occasionally it may be necessary to grade muscle strength. By carefully comparing the muscle groups of each limb, it is possible to detect any gross impairment. Muscle strength may be graded as follows:

0	No contracture on voluntary effort.
Poor	Ability to move the joint through full range of motion with gravity eliminated.
Fair	Power to move the joint through a full range of motion against gravity.
Good	Strength to move the joint against gravity plus some resistance.
Normal	Ability to move a joint through a full range of motion against good resistance (or the same resistance as on the "normal" side).

Muscle tightness may contribute to an exercise problem, particularly in the lower extremities. For example, in long-distance runners the gastro-soleus gradually tightens. The tightness of the gastrocnemius versus the soleus can be ascertained in the following manner. With the knee fully extended,

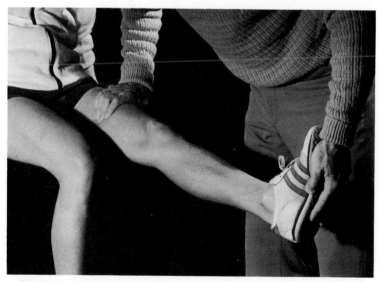

Fig 6–1.—Testing for tightness in the gastro-soleus group. Dorsiflexion of the foot is checked with the knee extended.

the gastrocnemius is under full tension. The foot is dorsiflexed and the range of motion noted. The same maneuver is repeated with the knee .flexed, which relaxes the gastrocnemius (Figs 6–1 and 6–2). Again, dorsiflexion is noted. Increased dorsiflexion with the knee flexed indicates tightness in the gastrocnemius muscle. If there is no change in dorsiflexion with the knee flexed, the tightness may be in either the gastrocnemius or the soleus. Hamstring tightness can be similarly ascertained by examining the patient supine, flexing the hip, first with the knee extended and then with the knee flexed.

Movement of the joints should be examined. There are two

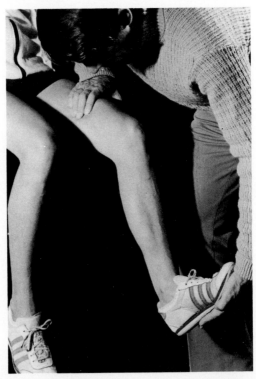

Fig 6–2.—Testing for tightness in the gastro-soleus group, step 2. The knee is flexed and dorsiflexion rechecked (see Fig 6–1). More dorsiflexion with the knee flexed indicates primary gastrocnemius contracture.

basic types of movement: passive (that movement which can be obtained by the examining physician) and active (that movement which the patient can accomplish).

Active movement should be examined, comparing the involved side with the uninvolved side, by asking the patient to flex, extend, abduct, adduct and rotate, depending on the joint. The American Academy of Orthopedic Surgeons manual, *Measuring and Recording of Joint Motion,* gives a standard normal range for individual variations. Memorization of motion tables is not necessary, however, because a normal side is available for comparison. Limitation of motion in all directions usually indicates a generalized condition such as arthritis. Limitation of motion in only 1 or 2 directions often indicates some type of mechanical problem. Active movement can be limited by pain, loss of muscle integrity, intrinsic joint stiffness or mechanical lesions within the joint.

Active motion should be compared with passive motion. The range of passive motion will exceed the range of active motion when the nerve to a muscle has been injured or when the muscle tendon unit has been disrupted. Increased motion at a joint indicates instability because of loss of integrity of ligaments, tendons, joint capsule or all 3.

Peripheral nerves can be damaged in athletic injuries. There are 3 types of trauma to nerves. Standard classification is as follows:

1. Neurotmesis — complete severence of a nerve, encountered in open wounds.
2. Axonotmesis — nerve tissue divided, nerve sheath intact, produced by compression or stretching of nerve.
3. Neurapraxia — nerve tissue and sheath intact, nerve has lost conductivity, mild compression of nerve tissue.

Fortunately, most nerve injuries are of the neurapraxic variety. In these injuries motor function is usually lost, but sensory function is retained. Spontaneous recovery of the motor function usually takes place within several days to several weeks, if the injured area is protected. It may be difficult in the early stages to differentiate a neurapraxia from an axonotmesis. The simplest test may be Tinel's test, performed by gently tapping over the area of injury. If paresthesias are pro-

TABLE 6-1.—COMMON NERVE ROOT SYNDROMES

LEVEL	SENSATION	MOTOR	REFLEX
C4-5 5th root	Anterolateral forearm	Scapula winged	Biceps depressed
C5-6 6th root	Thumb	Biceps weak	Biceps absent
C6-7 7th root	Index and long	Triceps weak	Triceps absent
C7-T1 8th root	Ring and little	Intrinsics weak	No changes
L3-4 4th root	Great toe	Quadriceps weak	Patellar absent
L4-5 5th root	Middle toes	Toe extensors weak	No changes
L5-S1 S1 root	Little toe	Plantar flexors weak	Ankle absent

duced, the nerve is probably in continuity. If no paresthesias are forthcoming, anatomical or physiologic severance of the nerve must be suspected. Electromyography or nerve conduction tests may be helpful in determining the severity of the nerve injury.

If there is no localized trauma but complaints of pain or loss of function are present, it is necessary to do a complete neurological examination. This examination is particularly important in those patients with back or neck problems. Common nerve root syndromes are given in Table 6-1.

RADIOLOGIC EXAM

Radiologic examination of the injured area should follow the physical exam. Many times the physician will think that an x-ray may not be indicated medically. Legally, this may not be the case. It is recommended that x-rays be obtained at the time of injury so that as much information as possible will be available before treatment.

It is advisable to order x-rays of the normal extremity, especially for children. A systematic method of viewing the x-ray should be followed. It is best to view the x-ray in the anatomical position on the viewbox. The general density of the bone should be noted, and any changes in the local density should be recognized. Margins of the bones should be examined in continuity and disruptions noted. Abnormal thickening or thinning of the cortex may be important. The joints should be aligned. Maintenance or absence of normal spaces and the overall appearance of the joint surfaces should be noted. The soft tissues should be inspected for localized swelling, calcifications or ossification. When there is a readily apparent problem, such as a fracture of a long bone, a complete evaluation of the film often is not done, causing the physician to miss an associated injury.

After viewing the routine films, special x-ray studies may be necessary. For joint problems, stress views may be helpful to determine the extent of injury to the ligamentous structures. Occasionally tomography, stereoscopic views or arthrography may be necessary.

After gathering all the above-mentioned data, a reasonably accurate diagnosis should be possible. Thus a rational treatment program can be developed.

GENERAL TREATMENT CONSIDERATIONS

Management of the orthopedic problems of athletes is divided into 3 different categories:
1. No specific treatment. The exam gives the athlete reassurance and confidence. Advice should be given that emphasizes prevention.
2. Nonoperative treatment.
3. Operative treatment.

Discussions of operative methods are not within the scope of this book. Problems that require surgery should be identified and the appropriate referral made.

Often the physician will not be able to give an exact diagnosis or a specific treatment, but the athlete will be comforted by a thorough examination and a discussion of the findings, or lack of them. The "treatment" in such cases is assurance that continued activity will not cause an irreversible problem.

In the following paragraphs, we will discuss the nonoperative treatment of athletic injuries, including immobilization, drugs, injections, modalities and therapy.

Immobilization

Many injuries and inflammations respond to rest. With most orthopedic problems, rest means immobilization of the injured area. In an emergency, a pillow, a folded magazine, a yardstick or a board may be all that is available, but any of these will certainly suffice. A compressive dressing to control swelling can be applied with a temporary splint. Following complete evaluation, a soft splint of felt or cast padding with an Ace bandage may be all that is necessary. More rigidity can be provided by a plaster splint. The most complete immobilization is obtained from a cast. Application of a cast requires training and practice. In chronic conditions braces are usually necessary. The degree and length of time of immobilization is dictated by the severity of the injury and its location.

Drugs

For most orthopedic problems no specific drug therapy is available. There is nothing yet to speed up the healing of bones or to decrease the severity of soft tissue injury. Most medications having any efficacy in orthopedic problems relieve pain, inflammation and muscle tightness.

The relief of pain is the primary interest of the patient. The exact cause of the pain must be determined. Once effective immobilization has been obtained, the requirements for analgesics are often reduced. The milder forms of pain medications, such as salicylates, are usually effective. The use of narcotics should be discouraged. Salicylates have additional effects on the blood coagulating mechanism and on the respiratory control centers. In addition to their analgesic properties, salicylates have an anti-inflammatory effect. However, like most anti-inflammatory medications, salicylates are gastric irritants. Therefore, because of their multisystem effects, unsupervised and continuous use of analgesics should not be allowed.

Antipyrine and aminopyrine, early anti-inflammatory agents, had so many side effects that they lost favor, both as analgesics and anti-inflammatory agents. The next anti-in-

TABLE 6-2.—ANTI-INFLAMMATORY AGENTS

TOXICITY	DRUG	DOSAGE°
Mild	Salicylates	600 mg q.i.d.
	Indomethacin	25-50 mg t.i.d. or q.i.d.
Moderate	Ibuproten	300-400 mg t.i.d. or q.i.d.
	Tolmetin Sodium	400 mg t.i.d.
	Naproxen	250 mg b.i.d. or t.i.d.
High	Oxyphenbutazone	100 mg t.i.d. or q.i.d.
	Phenylbutazone	100 mg t.i.d. or q.i.d.

°These are general dosages. Specific information should be obtained from package inserts.

flammatory agent, and a good one, to be developed was phenylbutazone. Because of its significant toxic side effects, mainly related to the gastrointestinal tract, it should not be used for more than 5-7 days. Oxyphenbutazone was introduced as a drug similar to phenylbutazone, but with less gastric irritation. In the past few years, several medicines have been developed that were supposedly less irritating to the intestine. They are indomethacin, tolmetrin sodium, naproxen and ibuprofen. Unfortunately, all these medications have variable gastric toxicity and must be prescribed with caution. They should all be taken after meals. Table 6-2 lists the different medications and their appropriate dosages.

Injections

In some joint injuries, injection of a local anesthetic into an injured area may be necessary to determine the extent of injury. With pain relief, and thus some relaxation of muscle guarding, it may be possible to determine more accurately the extent of ligamentous and capsular injury. This, however, should only be undertaken by the skilled, after a routine examination that is as complete as possible.

Some physicians advocate the injection of different enzymes into injured soft tissue or joints. For the same reason, others advocate oral enzymes to reduce bleeding, swelling and tissue damage. We have not found either oral or injectable enzymes to be efficacious in the management of athletic injuries.

There has been much discussion, most of it negative, on the use of injectable steroids. The use of steroids, either oral or injectable, should be limited to those patients with chronic rheumatoid arthritis or other forms of chronic disease managed by specialists. The intra-articular use of cortisone in the athlete is to be condemned. The powerful anti-inflammatory effect of cortisone and its derivatives removes the protective mechanism of the joint and makes it more susceptible to permanent damage.

Modalities

An acutely injured area has hemorrhage and swelling that must be controlled. The primary method of control is elevation, followed by the application of a compressive dressing and cold packs. Gentle treatment should be continued for 24 hours, possibly up to 48 hours, depending on the severity of the injury. If the application of cold increases the patient's discomfort, it should be discontinued.

After 48 hours the possibility of further bleeding into the injury site is minimal, provided there has been adequate immobilization. At this time it is safe to apply heat, which increases the local blood supply and speeds the healing process. Additionally, it relaxes the muscles, which may be in spasm secondary to the inflammation. Heat can be applied in several different forms. Dry heat can be administered with a standard heating pad. Moist heat can be administered either by a hydrocollator pack or by wrapping the injured area with a warm, moist towel covered in a plastic drape and held in place by an Ace bandage. Another method of applying wet heat is to wrap the injured area in a moist towel surrounded by a waterproofed heating pad. The most penetrating heat is administered by ultrasound.

Electrical stimulation is another modality that may be valuable. When an injured limb is immobilized for longer than several days, the muscle tissues begin to atrophy. Electrical stimulation causes the uncovered portion of the muscles to continue to contract, retarding the severity of atrophy. Small portable units for electrical stimulation can be given to the patient for treatment at home.

Therapy

Therapy is of 2 types, active or passive. Active therapy is performed by the patient, using the muscles available, putting the joint through as much motion range as possible. Passive therapy is done by someone else, with no participation on the patient's part. There is a third type, called active assistance, in which the patient activates the muscle carrying the joint through a range of motion as far as his strength will allow. The therapist assists in gently increasing the range. Active motion has 3 functions: to mobilize, to strengthen and to improve coordination. Passive motion mainly improves or preserves mobility.

When it is necessary to rest a joint to treat a particular problem, the joint will gradually become stiff. The safest way to regain that lost motion is by active exercise, which can usually be done by the patient. Occasionally the supervision of a trainer or therapist will be needed. In general, the athlete must regain a full range of functional motion before significant gains can be made in increasing muscle strength.

A muscle is strengthened by 2 forms of exercise. Muscle action without joint motion is called static exercise. Dynamic exercises are those which produce joint motion. Dynamic exercises are generally best because they increase both joint motion and strength.

There are 3 ways in which muscles contract: isotonically, isometrically, and eccentrically. An eccentric contraction is one in which the motion is produced by gravity, and the most efficient program is one which makes use of the principle of eccentric contractions. For example, to strengthen the biceps the athlete lifts a 20-pound barbell by moving the elbow from a completely extended position to a completely flexed position. If this maneuver takes 2 seconds, then the eccentric contraction, that is, returning the elbow to the completely extended position, should be doubled, or take 4 seconds. Repetitions like this increase the strength of the biceps more rapidly than if the elbow is allowed to be extended as quickly as possible. Similar eccentrically involved programs can be developed for each of the muscle groups by appropriate positioning of the extremity before the weight is lifted. It is not within the scope of this book to describe specific exercise programs for each group of muscles.

MUSCULOSKELETAL STRUCTURES

The musculoskeletal examination requires a basic knowledge and understanding of bones, joints, the musculotendinous unit and nerves. A brief review of the important elements of these structures will facilitate diagnosis and treatment.

Bone

Bone is a type of connective tissue composed of ground substance impregnated with deposits of calcium, phosphorus and other minerals. Cortical, or hard, bone generally surrounds softer, or cancellous, bone or may surround a space filled with marrow. There are two major bone types, flat and long. Additionally there is one specialized type of bone, the sesamoid, which is found within the tendon. A good example of the latter is the patella, situated within the quadriceps patellar tendon mechanism.

The processes of bone growth and fracture healing have several things in common. When bone is broken, a hematoma forms around the broken ends. The hematoma organizes into soft callous, which functions as the cartilage model. The soft callous becomes impregnated with calcium and other minerals, increasing in hardness. The hard callous gradually becomes bone, producing union.

Joints

A joint is a union between 2 bones. There are 3 large classifications of joints — fibrous, cartilaginous and synovial.

Fibrous joints are united by connective tissue. Because of the shapes of their articulating surfaces, there is often very little movement possible in these joints. Two examples of such a joint are the suture lines of the skull and the laminae of the vertebrae, which are held together by the ligamentum flava.

Cartilaginous joints are united by fibrocartilage instead of the usual hyaline cartilage. There is a small amount of movement present. Examples of this type are the pubic symphysis and the union between the vertebral bodies, which are separated by disks of fibrocartilage.

The most common type is a synovial joint (Fig 6–3). It is held together by ligaments but has smooth articulating surfaces of hyaline cartilage to allow movement. The 6 types of synovial joints, with examples of each, are listed below:

1. Ginglymus – the elbow and the interphalangeal joint
2. Trochoidal or pivot – the odontoid, and the proximal and distal radial ulnar articulations
3. Condyloid – the knee and the radial carpal joint
4. Saddle joint – first carpometacarpal joint
5. Cotylical or ball and socket joint – the shoulder and the hip joints
6. Plane – the acromioclavicular joints, and the intratarsal and intracarpal joints.

The typical cartilaginous joint is composed of several structures. The ends of the 2 bones involved in the joint are covered with hyaline cartilage, allowing them to move upon each other. The ends of the bones are held together by a fibrous structure called the joint capsule. Assisting in the sta-

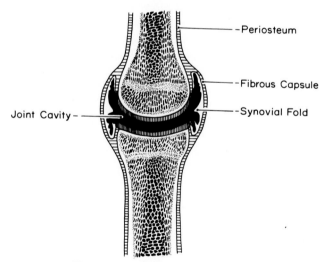

Fig 6–3. – A typical synovial joint.

bility of the joints are the ligaments. Lying on the inner layer of the joint capsule is a membrane composed of synovial tissue. All of that area surrounded by the synovial tissue is called the synovial cavity. The synovium secretes a fluid to lubricate and protect the hyaline cartilage. In injury, the synovial membrane produces excessive fluid to further protect the joint. Swelling produced by the excessive fluid stretches the joint capsule and ligaments, producing pain.

Muscles

Skeletal muscles are primarily voluntary muscles, containing their own nerves and their own blood supplies. The muscles are attached to bone by tendon in 2 areas. The area of attachment that is the least mobile is called the origin; the opposite mobile end is called the insertion. The origin and insertion of some muscles may vary, depending on which joint is fixed at a certain time in a period of motion. Usually the origin is the proximal end, and the insertion is the distal end. Anatomically, the insertion is always tendinous, whereas the origin may in some cases be muscular or fibrous.

Tendons are stronger structures than muscles. They are composed of nonliving fibers and are more capable of sustaining trauma than muscles. To protect muscles from underlying bony prominences, connective tissue pads are present. To protect the tendons from these same projections there are bursa and tendon sheaths. Fluid in the bursa provides a cushion to protect the tendon. Within the tendon sheath, a synovial-like fluid is produced to lubricate and allow the tendon to glide effortlessly. Trauma to the muscle or tendon increases the fluid in either of these spaces, causing pain and limitation of motion.

The strength of the muscle and the amount of movement the muscle can produce depends on several different factors: the actual number of muscle fibers being stimulated by the nerve, the position of the insertion at the time of activation, as well as the type of muscle.

Muscles contract in 3 ways. An isotonic or equal tension contracture is the shortening of a muscle fiber without great variation in the strength of the contraction; an isometric contraction is one in which opposing muscles work with equal strength but there is no movement of the part and thus no shortening of the muscle; an eccentric contraction occurs in a movement that can only be carried out by gravity. The muscles that oppose this movement must first contract and then gradually lengthen. Of the 3 types, eccentric contraction exercises are the most efficient in increasing strength.

Previously, muscles were classified according to their content of parallel, unipennate or bipennate fibers. This is not practical, as most muscles are a mixture. With improved techniques, particularly electromyography, it has been possible to identify muscles differently, according to their function in movement. Muscles are now categorized as prime movers or protagonists, synergists and antagonists. The prime mover is a muscle that produces a desired effect. A synergist is a muscle that contracts at the same time to potentiate the prime mover. The antagonist is a muscle that opposes the prime mover. In some instances there are no prime movers, as gravity provides this function. In this case the contracting muscle becomes the synergist.

Nerves

Every voluntary muscle is innervated by at least one nerve with several branches. The components of the one or several nerves are not always derived from the same spinal nerve. There may be two or more segmental levels of spinal localization involved in any one muscle. Destruction of any one peripheral nerve, or one spinal nerve, will not necessarily totally paralyze a whole muscle.

The typical nerve has both motor and sensory functions. The sensory portion of the nerve is concerned with many modalities other than pain. Most of the sensory impulses concerned with the muscles do not reach the level of consciousness. The nerve fibers coming from the muscle and those coming from the joint must coordinate in order to produce orderly motion. These are predominantly proprioceptive fibers, which are very important in learning skilled movement.

The motor nerve fibers to the muscle terminate on a motor end plate, which stimulates a certain muscle fiber. With that stimulation, an all-or-none contraction takes place within that fiber. The all-or-none principle does not apply to the total muscle, or such things as fine movements and gentle grasp would not be possible. Thus, voluntary movements can be modulated in strength and in speed. Training teaches one how to control these movements to provide skilled movement.

POINTS OF PHYSICAL EXAMINATION BY REGION AND REGIONAL PROBLEMS

Neck and Cervical Spine

The patient should be examined sitting on a stool or standing with the neck and upper torso bare. Inspection should take in the bony contours, the soft tissue contours, any scars or sinuses and the position of the head. Palpation should include the bony contours for comparison, right to left. Any soft tissue masses or areas of local tenderness should be noted. Motion exam includes flexion and extension of the cervical spine, lateral flexion to the right and left, and rotation. Note should be made of any pain or crepitation with movement. Longitudinal compression and traction should be applied to the cervical region to determine if pain is produced or relieved. A neurological examination of the upper extremities should be conducted, including testing of the various root levels for sensation, motor function and reflexes (see Table 6–1).

Cervical Strain

Cervical strain is a frequent problem seen in the office. Usually the athlete will have received some type of jolt that produced either acute flexion or acute extension of the neck. Often there is no particular discomfort during the first 24–72 hours. Then, nondescript soreness will develop, followed by stiffness. There may be radiation of the pain to the shoulders or into the arm. The athlete should be questioned about previous neck problems. Often there is some generalized tenderness in the cervical region and, occasionally, some muscle guarding. There may be some restriction of full neck motion, but neurological examination is usually normal. X-rays in the first-time episode will usually be normal. If there has been any previous history of problem there may be some narrowing of a disk space or some osteophyte formation.

The neck should be rested either by confining the patient to bed or by use of a soft cervical collar. The use of warm compresses, either moist or dry, is encouraged. A mild analgesic and a muscle relaxant can also be used. When there is marked muscle guarding or a list to one side, traction may be used. Traction can be prescribed in two forms: (1) over the end of the bed, using 8 – 10 pounds for 20 – 30 minutes, 3 or 4 times a day; or (2) over the door, again using the same weight for the same amount of time. Response to treatment is usually slow. If there has not been significant improvement in 10 – 14 days, the patient should be referred to a specialist.

Herniated Cervical Disk

In herniated cervical disk problems, the athlete complains of severe pain, usually more marked than with a strain. There may have been a flexion or extension injury followed by acute onset of pain that often radiates into the extremities. Frequently there is a history of neck problems. Physical examination usually reveals restricted motion, particularly on flexion and on turning to the painful side, and localized tenderness. Neurological examination should be performed to attempt localization of the disk level. X-rays should be obtained of the cervical spine, including obliques. The physician should look for narrowing of a particular disk space, osteophyte formation anteriorly on the margins of the body or posteriorly in the area of the foramen.

Treatment of the acute cervical disk is similar to that for a cervical sprain.

Spine and Back

The back should be fully unclothed from the neck to the gluteal area. The patient should be examined standing. Alignment of the spine is checked to determine if the normal lumbar lordosis and thoracic kyphosis is present. The presence of an uneven pelvis, a scoliosis or an increased kyphosis should be noted. Forward bending, the Adams position, will accentuate any spinal rotation with demonstration of a rib hump. Palpation should be done to determine any areas of tenderness or muscle guarding along the spine. Forward flexion, extension and lateral flexion should be observed. Splinting of the back without reversal of the normal lordosis on forward flexion should be noted. Neurological examination of the lower extremities should be done to isolate any root level problems (see Table 6–1).

Thoracic and Lumbar Spine

Differentiation of a lumbar strain from a lumbar disk problem is similar to that for the neck. Thoracic disks are rare, as are thoracic strains. The athlete complains of pain in the low back, often without radiation. In the more mature athlete there is increased likelihood of preexisting back disease. There may be some complaints of radiation of pain into the lower extremities. It is important to delineate the exact pain pattern. In most cases of either sprain or herniated disk the athlete is more comfortable when reclining than when either sitting or walking. Valsalva's maneuver, such as in coughing or sneezing, increases the discomfort, especially when there is a protuberant disk (Fig 6–4).

Examination will reveal some restriction of forward bending. The straight leg-raising test is positive, particularly if there is a disk herniation at L3-L4 or L5-S1. Pelvic rocking is

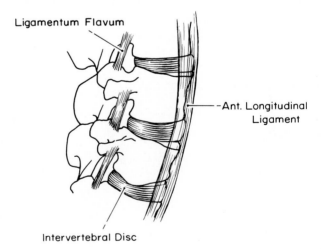

Fig 6–4.—Gross relationship in the lumbar spine. Spurring can occur anteriorly at the attachments of the anterior longitudinal ligament on the vertebral body. The disk can protrude posteriorly, pressing on the cord under the ligamentum flavum.

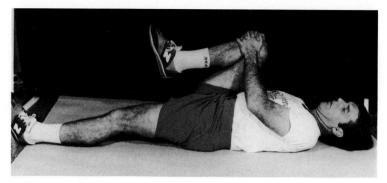

Fig 6–5. — The athlete lies on a flat surface and pulls one leg, then the other, up to the chest.

usually a more comfortable position unless significant osteoarthritis is present. The neurological examination is usually normal, but the more prolonged the symptoms the more likely there will be some aberration in either sensory, motor or reflex manifestations. X-rays should be obtained to delineate any significant disk space narrowing, any degenerative changes or any evidence of congenital malformation, such as spondylolysis or spondylolisthesis.

Treatment of either a strain or a herniated disk is the same at

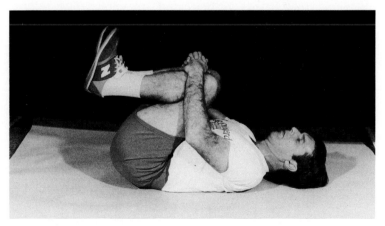

Fig 6–6. — The athlete pulls both knees up to the chest.

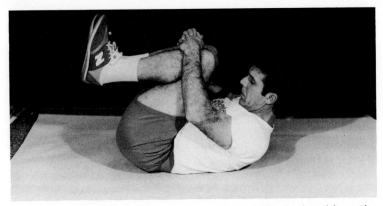

Fig 6–7.—The athlete pulls both knees and lifts the head from the surface simultaneously.

the outset. Usually bed rest is effective. Frequently the most comfortable position is a modified Fowler's position or the lounge-chair position, with the knees flexed about 30 degrees and the head elevated on a pillow 25–30 degrees. Analgesics, muscle relaxants and heat are prescribed. When the symptoms begin to subside, exercises should be instituted (Figs 6–5 to 6–9). Each exercise should be done in sets of 10, 3 or 4 times daily for 4 weeks. If the symptoms do not resolve and there is suspicion that a disk is herniated, an appropriate referral should be made.

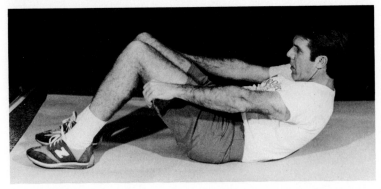

Fig 6–8.—The athlete performs situps with the knees bent.

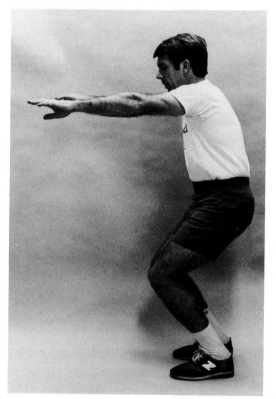

Fig 6–9.—The athlete stands with his back straight, does a slow squat, holds for 20 sec, then rapidly returns to a standing position.

Shoulder

The patient should be examined in a standing position from both back and front. Asymmetries of the muscles or posture abnormalities should be noted. Palpation of the bony prominences, particularly over the anterior superior aspect of the shoulder and the acromioclavicular joint, should be done to determine any localized tenderness or swelling. Movements (both active and passive) to be tested are abduction, flexion, extension, and internal and external rotation. The examiner's hand should be placed gently on the shoulder joint to perceive any crepitus or winging of the scapula. Note whether the scapulothoracic and glenohumeral motions are taking place in a synchronous manner by comparing motions on the opposite side. Normally, about half the motion is glenohumeral and half is scapular rotation. The two motions can be separated by trapping the inferior border of the scapula in one hand and asking the patient to abduct the shoulder. This should allow abduction to about 80 or 90 degrees. Releasing the scapula should allow full range of motion. The examination should include testing the power of the shoulder abductors, arm flexors and rotators of the shoulder.

Painful Shoulder Syndrome

Painful shoulder is a common complaint among athletes, particularly as age advances. The pain occasionally extends into the upper arm when the shoulder has been abducted from 45 degrees to 120 degrees. There is usually no pain with full abduction or with the arm completely at rest at the side. This syndrome can be produced by several different lesions, all of which cause pain by trapping a tender structure between the acromion process and the tuberosity of the humerus. The distance between these two bony prominences is the least between 45 and 145 degrees of abduction.

Several problems involving the supraspinatus tendon can create pain. A minor tear of the supraspinatus tendon can cause pain without loss of power. A calcium deposit within the supraspinatus tendon will become surrounded by an inflammation (Fig 6 – 10), which takes up space and causes impingement through the arc of abduction. This particular cause is often acute and can be extremely uncomfortable. Another lesion of the supraspinatus tendon is an inflammation secondary to degeneration of tendon fibers. The fourth cause of pain in this area is an incomplete fracture of the tuberosity of the humerus or contusion of the bony prominence of the humerus. All create swelling that obliterates the acromiohumeral space with abduction. Primary inflammation and swelling of the subacromial bursa, which occupies this small space, is another cause. another cause.

It is often difficult for even the experienced examiner to differentiate the exact etiology of the pain. Only with calcifica-

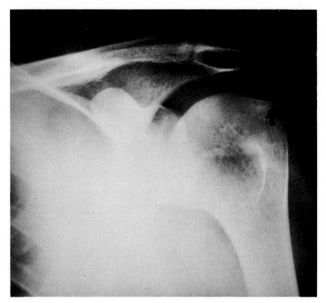

Fig 6–10. — Calcific bursitis of the shoulder with surrounding sclerotic reaction.

tion of the supraspinatus tendon is the diagnosis correctly identified. For this reason, x-rays of the shoulder should be obtained.

Initial treatment of all these entities is similar. The shoulder should be immobilized in a sling. Heat should be provided by hot packs, hydrocolators or ultrasound. Mild analgesics are often necessary. Symptoms will generally subside with this treatment unless there is a significant calcium deposit. With this, the pain is often so intense and the patient so uncomfortable that something more vigorous needs to be done. Aspirating the calcium deposits with a large needle can be tried. Often aspiration is unsuccessful, but the needle may rupture the surrounding bursal sac, thus relieving some of the discomfort. This is one of the few instances where an injection of cortisone may be indicated to reduce inflammation. In chronic shoulder problems caused by any of these entities, a partial acromionectomy may be necessary.

Rotator Cuff Tear

The rotator cuff, composed of the supraspinatus, infraspinatus, subscapularis and teres minor, is mainly involved in elevating and abducting the shoulder (Fig 6–11). Cuff tears are more common in mature athletes. Usually there is some preexisting fraying of the cuff, secondary to use. A sudden force, such as might be encountered in tackling or lifting weights, creates a tear. The athlete will complain of pain in the shoulder, particularly when it is abducted to about 90 degrees. There will be difficulty performing any activities with the hand above the head, but there is little discomfort below that level. The athlete may also complain of pain when turning over on the shoulder at night and often adopts a position of sleeping away from the painful shoulder. Examination of the athlete with a complete tear demonstrates a tender area over the anterior superior aspect of the shoulder. If the arm is abducted to 90 degrees and then let go, the patient will not be able to maintain the shoulder in that position. The arm will drop to about 30 degrees, when control is then possible. Active abduction will not be possible beyond 30–45 degrees.

Treatment of acute rotator cuff rupture in the younger patient

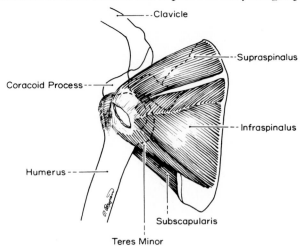

Fig 6–11.—A tear of the rotator cuff usually occurs in the tendon of the supraspinatus.

should be surgical. In the older patient, where there is fraying of the tendon or if the athlete is seen several days past acute onset, the arm should be immobilized in a sling for 3 weeks. Range-of-motion exercises of increasing difficulty are started, and strengthening exercises for the shoulder muscles are added as motion improves. Most athletes will get well, but some do not. In that instance the choice must be made either to stop those activities which the patient cannot do or to consider surgery. Surgical correction is not uniformly successful. It may relieve the discomfort without restoring full function. A shoulder arthrogram may be valuable preoperatively.

Subluxing Biceps Tendon (Snapping Shoulder)

Athletes involved in sports that require throwing may complain of shoulder snapping. Frequently, a subluxation of the biceps tendon is the cause. The problem is produced when the covering of the bicipital groove is torn. Examination usually reveals tenderness in the biceps groove. With the arm in internal rotation, tenderness is medial and, if the arm is externally rotated, the tenderness moves laterally. A test for this problem is performed as follows: The examiner grasps the flexed elbow with one hand and holds the wrist with the other (Fig 6–12). The arm is slowly rotated externally and the elbow extended at the same time. If this creates pain, it indicates a problem in the bicipital groove. If the tendon is unstable, it will pop out of the groove and the patient will experience immediate pain. X-rays, particularly tangential views of the shoulder, often demonstrate an abnormality of the groove, which may be too shallow, allowing the tendon to slide back and forth. The tendon will only dislocate if the covering of the groove has been ruptured.

By the time the patient is seen and a subluxing or dislocating biceps tendon is diagnosed, the problem is chronic. The nonsurgical approach is to abstain from throwing or weight lifting. If this is not acceptable for the athlete, surgical correction will be necessary.

Adhesive Capsulitis (Frozen Shoulder)

Many inflammatory conditions previously discussed can lead to generalized inflammation within the glenohumeral joint. However, there is an ill-defined and not fully under-

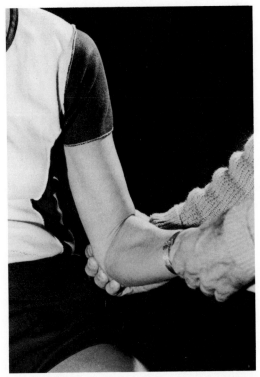

Fig 6–12.—To test for subluxing of the long biceps tendon, grasp the patient's flexed elbow with one hand, rotate the arm externally and pull down on the elbow. If the tendon is unstable, it will dislocate from the bicipital groove, causing pain.

stood entity that occurs in older athletes. Any problem previously discussed regarding the shoulder joint may precipitate capsulitis, or it may occur without any predisposing factor. Usually the athlete is over 40 and complains of generalized pain in the shoulder and loss of motion. Pain may be present for a number of months. During that time, motion is gradually lost until very little remains. X-rays are usually normal.

After a number of months the pain gradually subsides. During this time rest in a sling for short periods may help. Maintenance of as much shoulder motion as possible is encouraged by prescribing circumduction and pendulum exercises. As the pain lessens, active exercises are intensified. Fortunately, the problem is self-limiting and gradually improves. Anti-inflammatory agents, injections or manipulations do not usually alter the pathologic process. The patient should be informed that it is going to take a long time to get well. In the author's experience, these patients uniformly become pain-free and usually regain almost normal function.

Chronic Dislocation of the Shoulder

A shoulder that has been dislocated more than once is termed chronic. Acute dislocation is discussed in Chapter 7. X-rays should be obtained to identify the dislocation as anterior, posterior or subglenoid. This is an important point when considering an operative repair. The neurologic examination should include testing the sensory distribution of the axillary nerve over the lateral border of the shoulder.

After x-rays have been obtained, reduction can be accomplished by applying traction in the long axis of the shoulder muscles. The shoulder should be immobilized in a sling in internal rotation for 3 weeks and range-of-motion exercises begun at the conclusion. Then strengthening exercises for the rotator cuff muscles, the deltoid and the biceps are prescribed. Usually after a second dislocation and certainly after a third, surgery should be considered.

Subluxation of the Shoulder

Subluxation may occur anteriorly, inferiorly or posteriorly, the most common being anterior. There is usually a history of injury that has forced the humeral head against the anterior joint capsule and torn it. The athlete says that he felt as if his shoulder had slipped out at some time in the past. The shoulder was spontaneously reduced, followed by soreness for a day or so. Gradually use is resumed. After the initial episode there may be feelings of instability about the shoulder joint.

If the problem is not more than several weeks to several months old, immobilization with a sling, holding the arm internally rotated and fixed to the side, may allow the capsular structures to tighten. This is followed by mobilization and strengthening exercises for the shoulder musculature. However, because this diagnosis is often subtle, especially when the problem is an inferior or posterior subluxation, diagnosis may be difficult and treatment even more so. It is probably safest to refer patients with a complaint of instability to an orthopedic surgeon.

Acromioclavicular Joint Separation

The unrecognized acromioclavicular joint separation may become painful. If the joint capsule is only partially torn or, in the well-muscled individual, completely torn but unrecognized, the scarring and instability may produce shoulder discomfort, particularly in throwing activities. Examination reveals tenderness over the acromioclavicular joint. In a third-degree injury there will be a stepoff noted with abnormal motion in the clavicle upon depression. Routine x-rays of the shoulder may not show the pathology, and it is often necessary to take a standard anterior view of the acromioclavicular joint. Another anterior view with the athlete holding a 10-pound weight in his hand will accentuate any marginal stepoff.

If the athlete is seen within 10–14 days after injury, immobilization in a sling for a week to 10 days followed by gradual resumption of exercises may be all that is indicated. Many will have satisfactory shoulder function, except for a pitcher or a quarterback. After 14 days, it is probably too late for an open reduction and repair. Likewise, it is too early to excise the distal end of the clavicle. Referral to an orthopedist is probably the safest course.

Arm and Elbow

The bony and muscular contours should be noted with the elbow extended amd flexed. The angle the elbow makes in full extension should be noted. Normally, this angle—the carrying angle—is about 10 degrees of valgus. This angle can be lost in certain elbow fractures, especially those occurring in childhood.

Elbow Problems

Lateral Epicondylitis (Tennis Elbow)

Inflammation in the region of the lateral epicondyle at the origin of the supinator muscles is a common problem. It is frequently, but not exclusively, seen in tennis players. It is thought that the cause is overuse of an inadequately conditioned muscle group. The athlete, usually active only on weekends, will complain of pain over the lateral epicondyle of the humerus when shaking hands, twisting a doorknob or performing any activity that requires gripping. Examination reveals tenderness that often extends distally over the radial head in the extensor-supinator muscle mass. Resistance applied to wrist extension will re-create the pain at the elbow.

Lateral epicondylitis in a tennis player is thought to be produced by one or a combination of conditions: too large or too small a racket grip, racket strings either too tight or too loose or an improper stroke, particularly the backhand. Probably the primary cause is playing too much tennis too early in the season or playing significantly more tennis in a day than one normally plays. Questioning the patient usually brings out one or a combination of these factors. This is important, as the patient frequently will have a recurrence if the cause is not understood.

Treatment can be difficult. The best method is rest, even to the extent of placing the arm in a cast. However, most weekend athletes usually will not accept this. They have heard that an injection of cortisone into the area produces the quickest and surest cure; thus, many patients request it. If the patient decides on injections, a small-gauge needle should be used to infiltrate the area with a local anesthetic. The author prefers to mix a cortisone preparation with xylocaine and inject the two simultaneously. The athlete should be warned that the arm may hurt more for the first 12–24 hours following the injection. After relief of symptoms, the athlete usually starts playing too soon. There should be a period of forearm-strengthening exercises, such as gripping a ball, play dough or similar substance, before play is resumed. Another exercise involves lifting a 5-lb weight, using the wrist extensors, for several weeks before resuming activity. In refractory cases, injecting the elbow and immobilizing in a cast has proved helpful. Even under the best of circumstances, some athletes will not respond to treatment and surgery may be necessary.

Medial Epicondylitis (Golfer's Elbow)

Inflammation of the flexor pronator group of muscles at their origin on the medial epicondyle of the humerus is much less frequent than lateral epicondylitis. Symptoms are similar, and the physical findings likewise are similar. The only real difference from lateral epicondylitis is that the medial epicondyle lies immediately in front of the ulnar nerve. Occasionally the inflammation may be extensive enough to irritate the ulnar nerve. The athlete may complain of paresthesias in the distribution of the ulnar nerve. Tapping over the nerve may elicit a positive Tinel's test.

Treatment is similar to that for lateral epicondylitis. One must remember, when injecting the lateral epicondylar area, that the ulnar nerve is in close proximity. The needle should be kept a safe distance from it. The patient should be warned that there may be numbness in the distribution of the ulnar nerve associated with some weakness of the hand muscles for a period following injection. As the symptoms subside, the athlete should be instructed to do forearm-strengthening exercises as mentioned above.

Olecranon Bursitis

The bursa overlying the tip of the olecranon is frequently injured by direct trauma. The acute injury is often overlooked. Sometime later the athlete realizes that there is a painless swelling over the tip of the elbow. There is no loss of motion. X-rays are usually normal except for the soft tissue swelling. Occasionally in an acute case there may be a chip of the olecranon. In a chronic case there may be some calcifications within the bursal area.

Whether the condition is acute or chronic, the bursal sac should be aspirated. A small amount of cortisone is injected into the sac and a compression dressing applied. Frequently the fluid will reaccumulate, and subsequent injections may be necessary. Repeated injuries to this area may cause the bursa to become so thickened that only surgical excision will solve the problem.

Ulnar Nerve Contusion (Crazy Bone)

Because of the close proximity of the ulnar nerve to the skin as it courses behind the medial epicondyle at the elbow, it is frequently subject to injury. When the nerve is contused, tingling occurs distally. This may cause some dysfunction in the nerve for several days to several weeks. Examination reveals tenderness in the ulnar groove. Tapping over the ulnar nerve in the groove gives a positive Tinel's test. In extreme cases there may be a weakness of the intrinsic muscles of the hand.

Usually the contusion responds to rest in a sling, with *no* pressure applied posterior to the medial epicondyle. Injections and anti-inflammatory agents are usually not effective. If the nerve area remains tender and Tinel's test is positive, anterior transplantation of the nerve may be necessary.

Sprains and Strains of the Elbow

The elbow is a very stable joint powered by the strong biceps in flexion and the strong triceps in extension. Because of this, sprains and strains are uncommon injuries, even in the most violent of sports. When they do occur, the symptoms and findings will be similar to those of other joint injuries, depending on whether they are first, second or third degree.

Treatment depends upon the severity of the sprain. Fortunately, third-degree sprains or strains are relatively uncommon. First- and second-degree injuries usually respond to rest.

Forearm and Wrist

Inspection, with both arms bare, reveals malalignment, soft tissue swelling or discoloration. Palpation of the bony contours and the soft tissues delineates areas of tenderness or swelling. Examination of the anatomical snuff box located at the base of the thumb, between the extensor and abductors of the thumb, is important in wrist pain problems, for tenderness in this area often indicates injury to the carpal navicular. Radiocarpal joint motion is checked for flexion, extension, abduction and adduction. Supination and pronation motion indicates function of the radioulnar joints. Stability of the joint should be checked and the strength of the flexors, extensors, supinators and pronators should be graded.

Stenosing Tenosynovitis (deQuervain's Disease)

Pain on the radial side of the wrist without a history of injury may be caused by stenosing tenosynovitis. The short extensor tendon and the abductor tendon to the thumb pass through a tunnel across the radial styloid on their way to the base of the thumb. With overuse of either the thumb or the wrist, these tendons may become inflamed, producing a space problem within the tunnel. Thus motion of the thumb or wrist will create pain. Examination reveals tenderness and swelling. Finkelstein's test, performed by fully flexing the thumb and ulnar deviating the wrist, is positive.

Overuse must be stopped by immobilizing the wrist and thumb in a thumb spica. Injection of the tunnel with a local anesthetic and small amount of steroids is often effective. During injection, care should be taken not to enter the bodies of the tendon, as this may cause a roughened area on the tendon that prolongs the irritation. Resistant problems can be cured by surgically releasing the tendons from the tunnel.

Carpal Tunnel Syndrome

An athlete with carpal tunnel syndrome will complain of pain in the arm and hand, which is frequently worse at night. There is usually associated tingling and numbness in the hand

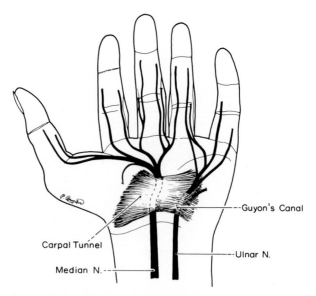

Fig 6–13.—Compression of the median nerve in the carpal tunnel causes symptoms of carpal tunnel syndrome. Occasionally pressure occurs on the ulnar nerve in Guyon's canal. Tapping the nerve over the canal may reproduce the symptoms.

in the distribution of the median nerve, which runs from the forearm into the hand underneath the transverse carpal ligament (Fig 6–13). In this same limited space are 8 flexor tendons to the fingers and the long flexor to the thumb. Any condition that decreases this space will cause compression of the median nerve. Direct trauma from falling on the wrist, fracture of the wrist, carpal bone dislocation, ganglion or synovitis of the flexor tendons from overuse can all cause symptoms. Examination in the early stages may be negative. Later there may be a positive Tinel's sign obtained by tapping over the nerve proximal to the carpal tunnel. Phalen's test, performed by having the patient make a fist and flex the wrist for a minute, may produce numbness and tingling in the distribution of the nerve. There may be weakness of the thenar musculature and decreased sensation in the distribution of the median nerve, sparing all of the fifth finger and half of the ring finger.

Immobilization in a wrist splint or a short arm cast to reduce the irritation in the carpal tunnel can be effective. If immobilization does not relieve the symptoms in several days, an injection of cortisone is often curative. In the refractory case a surgical release of the tunnel may be necessary.

Ulnar Nerve Entrapment

The ulnar nerve passes through Guyon's canal at the ulnar side of the wrist (see Fig 6–12). The condition is similar to a carpal tunnel syndrome except that the ulnar nerve is involved. The athlete complains of pain along the base of the fifth finger with paresthesias of the fifth and ring fingers. In a long-standing problem there may be atrophy of the hypothenar musculature.

The wrist should be immobilized in a splint. If the symptoms do not subside in a short period of time, an injection of cortisone can be tried. Care must be taken to avoid injuring the immediately adjacent ulnar artery. Occasionally surgical decompression of the nerve is necessary.

Ganglion

The most frequent location of a ganglion is the dorsoradial aspect of the wrist. This may not be a true sports injury. However, the athlete often has sustained a sprain of the wrist. The ganglion may have been present for some time but contained entirely within the wrist joint capsule. The minor injury may produce enough weakness in the joint capsule to allow herniation of the ganglion between the extensor tendons. Examination reveals a fluctuant mass that is usually fixed but may be movable. X-rays are usually negative.

If the ganglion is seen within the first several weeks of its appearance, it may rupture spontaneously. It should be given an opportunity to do so. If the ganglion has been present for several months, rupture by careful aspiration and injection of a small amount of cortisone has been about 50% effective in the author's hands. If this treatment fails, surgical excision should be done. Excision by the inexperienced surgeon is attended by a high recurrence.

Wrist Sprain

Wrist sprains are a common problem seen in the office. The usual cause is falling on the outstretched hand. Several hours later the wrist becomes swollen and tender. Most of the time the athlete will wait several days before deciding to seek medical attention. By this time, a first-degree sprain will feel better and thus may never be seen in the office. In the second-degree sprain there will be marked swelling and tenderness over the wrist joint with no instability. If instability is present, there has been a complete tear of one of the carpal or intercarpal ligaments. Recently a number of carpal disassociation syndromes have been described. These syndromes are produced by tears of individual intercarpal ligaments, producing instability of one or more of the carpal bones. Both physical and x-ray findings are very subtle.

The second-degree sprained wrist should be immobilized in a splint or cast for 3 weeks. A third-degree injury probably requires surgical repair. After 3 weeks' immobilization, if tenderness and swelling are still present, a disassociation syndrome should be suspected and the patient referred for orthopedic consultation. In the disassociation syndromes, early surgery produces the best results.

Hand

The bony alignment and the appearance of the soft tissue should be noted in examining the hand. Palpation of the thenar eminence reveals any absence of muscle tone or soft tissue swelling. The carpal tunnel area should be examined by tapping over the tunnel to see if paresthesias are produced in the median nerve distribution. Guyon's canal, which houses the ulnar nerve, should be examined similarly. Movement of joint, flexion, extension, abduction and adduction should be checked. The strength of the muscles that make those movements should be graded. The strength and individual motions of the flexor digitorium profundus and sublimis should be examined for each finger. Neurological examination of the hand includes median, ulnar and radial nerve function (Fig 6–14). The location of sensation for the radial nerve is in the

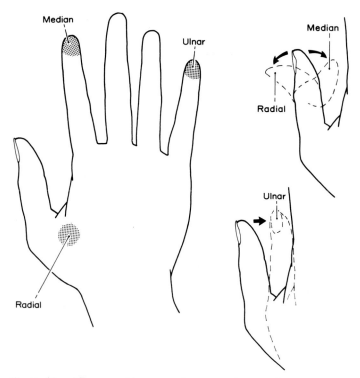

Fig 6–14.—A reasonably accurate evaluation of nerve function in the upper extremity can be done using the thumb for the motor indicator and the constant areas for sensory function.

web between the thumb and index finger and, for the ulnar nerve, in the tip of the fifth finger. The motor examination of all 3 nerves can be done with the thumb. Extension of the thumb is radial nerve function, flexion of the thumb is the medial nerve and adduction of the thumb is the ulnar nerve.

Hand and Finger Problems

Management of fractures in the hand and fingers is discussed in Chapter 7.

Stenosing Tenosynovitis (Trigger Finger)

Trigger finger is not a common injury in athletes, but occasionally it is seen. The athlete complains that full flexion causes the finger to "catch." It will not straighten out except by passive, painful manipulation. The athlete frequently localizes his problem to the level of the proximal interphalangeal joint. Examination reveals that full motion is present but, with either active or passive full flexion of the joint, the tendon catches and full extension is impossible. Once the finger has been extended, the athlete may complain of pain along the volar aspect near the proximal phalanx. Palpation reveals tenderness at the distal palmar crease. Occasionally a nodule can be felt.

The only nonoperative treatment is injection of the tendon sheath with a small amount of cortisone. This usually cures; but if it fails, surgical release of the tendon sheath is necessary.

Paronychia (Runaround)

An abrasion around the base of the nail anywhere on the cuticle may become infected. When this occurs the infection burrows underneath the cuticle area, creating a closed-space abscess. If this occurs at the base of the nail, pressure of the abscess may interfere with the germinal matrix and cause nail death.

In the early stages, warm soaks 2–4 times a day for 10 or 20 minutes may prevent abscess formation. If an abscess forms, the cuticle area should be lifted with a blunt instrument to allow the abscess to decompress. If this is unsuccessful, an incision should be made parallel to the long axis of the nail at the base and the flap lifted. Occasionally involvement may be so severe that the nail will have to be removed. Following decompression of the abscess and/or removal of the nail, warm compresses should be continued. Only in rare cases will the nail not grow back.

Felon

An abscess located within the pulp of the fingertip is called a felon. Because the space is small and tight, a very small amount of pus may create a large swelling and severe pain. If the pressure goes unrelieved, involvement of the distal phalanx may occur, causing osteomyelitis.

The abscess must be incised and drained through an incision on either the ulnar or the radial border of the fingertip. A small drain should be left in place for several days, and then warm soaks should be started.

Joint Instability

Instability of finger or thumb joints occasionally occurs following dislocation. The athlete usually says that he had a finger out of joint that was replaced by himself or by the trainer; no further treatment was received. In such an injury, instability will be noticed within a short period of time. The athlete complains that he cannot pinch or grasp as he previously could. The most commonly injured joints are the proximal interphalangeal joint of the index or fifth fingers and the metacarpal phalangeal joint of the thumb. Examination usually reveals swelling of the involved joint. Palpation may reveal tenderness in the region of the collateral ligament on the side of the swelling. Normally full range of flexion and extension are possible, but there is abnormal motion with either radial or ulnar stress of the joint. The stress may also be painful. X-rays should be obtained to rule out a fracture.

If the injury is seen within 2–3 weeks of onset, a period of splinting may allow healing of this third-degree ligament injury. Immobilization should continue for 3 weeks and then gradual mobilization begun. If the injury is older than 3 weeks and the instability is a significant problem, surgery will be necessary.

Tendon Rupture

Contact sports occasionally will produce tendon ruptures. The most frequently ruptured tendon is the profundus, usually of the index or the middle finger. The athlete may remember something happening to his finger but may not notice that it does not function well until a day or so later. He will complain that he cannot bend the finger fully. Examination reveals that the flexor digitorium sublimus is intact but that full flexion at the distal interphalangeal joint is not possible. X-rays should be obtained but usually are not helpful.

If the rupture is seen within a week to 10 days, the tendon can be repaired primarily. If several weeks have passed, a delayed procedure involving a tendon graft will be necessary.

Pelvis and Hip

The athlete is first examined standing and then walking. Note is taken whether the pelvis is level. An unlevel pelvis can be due to a short leg or to a pelvic obliquity brought on by a muscular or spinal disorder. The athlete's gait and stride length should be observed. Observation of the athlete in the sitting position is also necessary. A patient will sit lightly on a painful hip. Palpation demonstrates areas of tenderness or swelling. Particular attention should be paid to the posterior gluteal area, where the sciatic nerve exits from the pelvis. The greater trochanter area should be examined for tenderness. Leg length should be measured as previously described (see p. 84). Pressure should be applied over both iliac crests to test for any sacroiliac joint problems. Hip flexion, extension, abduction, adduction and rotation should be checked. The strength of the major muscle groups should be graded. Hip flexion deformity is checked with the patient supine. One hip is flexed fully and the position of the opposite hip is noted. It should lie on the examining table. If it flexes, the degree of flexion is the fixed flexion deformity. The test is repeated for the opposite hip.

Bursitis of the Hip

Falling on, or being hit upon, the greater trochanter of the femur (Fig 6–15) may cause inflammation of the greater tro-

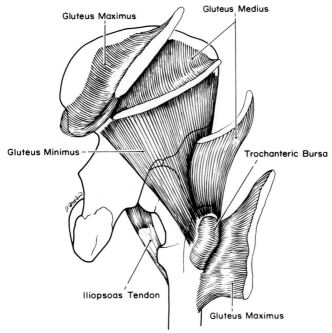

Fig 6–15.—The major muscles around the hip and their relationship to the pelvis and femur.

chanteric bursa. Such an injury is followed by pain and occasionally by swelling. Examination occasionally reveals an antalgic gait, in which a short step is taken on the painful side. X-rays should be obtained, but are usually normal.

In a fresh injury (that is, within 24–48 hours), ice should be applied and analgesics given. After 72 hours, heat in the form of hot compresses or whirlpool baths should be started. This will take care of the problem most of the time. If not, anti-inflammatory agents may be tried. If the oral agents fail, steroid injection into the bursa is usually effective.

Iliac Contusion (Hip Pointer)

Contusion of the iliac crest, avulsion of the muscles attaching to the crest or even a fracture of the pelvic rim produces pain along the crest of the ilium. The athlete complains that he cannot run without pain; in fact, he may not be able to run at all.

Initially the area should be treated with ice packs. If discomfort is severe, indicating significant muscle detachment, strapping of the area with tape may be necessary. When the athlete can run without limping, he can return to sports, with the iliac crest area well padded. Strapping should continue for 6–8 weeks.

Snapping or Clicking Hip

Following contusion to the greater trochanteric area, the athlete may complain that his hip snaps or slips out when it is in certain positions. Often this is not painful but merely bothersome. On examination, with flexion of the hip, the click may be palpated over the greater trochanter. This probably represents the iliotibial band or the gluteus muscles moving back and forth over the bony prominence of the trochanter.

Reassurance as to what the problem is, and that functionally it will not create any problems, is usually all that is required. If the snapping seriously bothers the athlete, surgery may be necessary.

Stress Fracture of the Pelvis or Hip

With so many people becoming involved in long-distance running, stress fractures are often showing up in the lower extremities. If a runner complains of pain in the pubic area or in the hip area not associated with tenderness or swelling or any other physical findings, a stress fracture must be suspected. If the injury is less than 3 or 4 weeks old, x-rays may be negative (Figs 6–16 and 6–17).

Iliopsoas Tendinitis

Tendinitis of the iliopsoas tendon at its insertion on the lesser trochanter is occasionally seen. The athlete complains of pain in the hip but is vague about its localization. Often there is no history of injury. Examination reveals some deep tenderness over the joint area. If the athlete is asked to flex his hip against resistance with the knee bent, the symptoms may be reproduced. X-rays are usually not helpful.

The inflamed area is so deep within the muscle mass that cold or heat usually will not penetrate. Rest is necessary, even

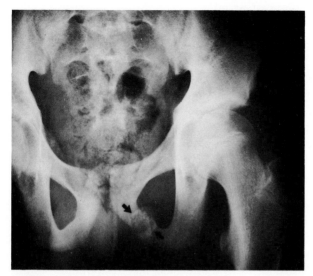

Fig 6–16. – X-ray of a 16-year-old cross-country runner with 3-month history of pain in the left hip.

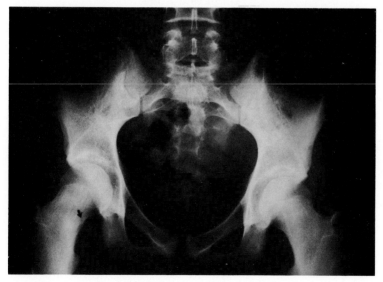

Fig 6–17. – X-ray of 18-year-old runner with 8-week history of a limp and pain in the right hip.

to the point of using crutches. Anti-inflammatory agents are used. Aspirin is tried first, and if it is ineffective one of the stronger anti-inflammatory agents can be used (see Table 6–2). It may take several weeks for the inflammation to clear.

Adductor Strain (Groin Pull)

Adductor strain may occur with a maximal effort, such as tackling or blocking in football. It may be caused by jumping if the athlete fails to warm up properly. Examination reveals tenderness along the adductor muscles in the groin region. There is usually very little swelling. An antalgic gait often is present.

If the injury is seen early, ice should be applied for the first 24–48 hours. Analgesics are often helpful. After 72 hours, heat, either from moist compresses or whirlpool baths, should be administered. Occasionally anti-inflammatory agents will be helpful. The athlete should not be allowed to return to activity until all local tenderness has disappeared and until he can run without a limp.

Thigh and Knee

In thigh and knee problems, the athlete should be examined walking, sitting, and going up and down steps. Inspection will reveal any disalignment of the extremity. The relationship of the patella, the insertion of the patellar tendon and the foot to a line from the anterior superior iliac spine to the floor should be noted. Another important relationship is the Q angle, determined by drawing one line along the longitudinal axis of the femur through the center of the patella and another line from the center of the insertion of the patellar tendon through the center of the patella. The angle created by the intersection of these two lines should not be greater than 10 degrees. A larger angle indicates malalignment of the extension mechanism of the knee and may be meaningful in patellar pain problems.

Palpation will pinpoint areas of tenderness, swelling or soft tissue masses. The motion of the patella on the femur should be checked with the knee fully extended and the quadriceps relaxed. The patella is displaced proximally, distally, medially, and laterally and the undersurface palpated to detect crepitus or roughness. Apley's test for subpatellar problems is performed with the quadriceps mechanism relaxed, the patella is displaced distally, and the athlete is instructed to activate the quadriceps. If there is any significant roughness of the patellar cartilage, pain may be produced.

Another common area of tenderness around the knee is that along the medial proximal surface of the tibia, where the pes anserine bursa is located. Frequently, the inferior pole of the patella is tender at the insertion of the patellar tendon on the tibial tubercle. Knee flexion and extension and the strength of these movements should be checked.

Stability of the ligaments must be tested. The collateral ligaments are tested with the knee fully extended. The medial ligament is tested by applying a valgus stress, the lateral ligament by applying a varus stress (Fig 6–18). The contribution of the joint capsule to stability can be removed by flexing the knee approximately 15 degrees and retesting with valgus and varus strain. If there is severe or third-degree ligament damage, the joint will open on the side of the damaged ligament. If stress causes pain but not instability, the ligament is probably

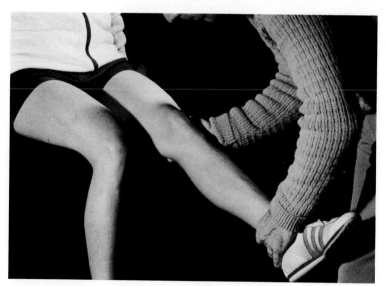

Fig 6–18.—To test the medial collateral ligament, pressure is applied at the knee laterally and at the ankle medially.

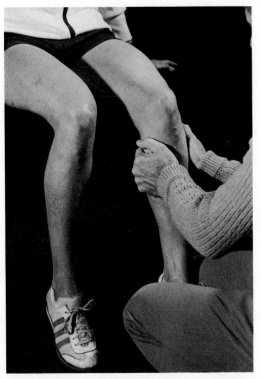

Fig 6–19.—Anterior-posterior laxity, when pressure is applied at the knee, indicates a torn cruciate ligament.

partially or completely intact. The cruciate ligaments are tested by looking for the "drawer sign" (Fig 6–19). The test is performed with the patient in the sitting position. The examiner grasps the patient's ankle between his knees and pulls anteriorly on the proximal fibula to test the anterior cruciate. Posterior pressure is applied to test the posterior cruciates. There should be no movement if both ligaments are intact.

The menisci are examined by MacMurray's test, performed with the patient sitting with the knee flexed. The examiner extends and externally rotates the tibia on the femur (Fig 6–20). Complaints of pain can be significant, as can a painful click. The pain produced by a torn cartilage can often be differentiated from capsular or ligamentous pain with Apley's test, which is performed with the patient prone. The leg is elevated by grasping the ankle and the leg is rotated (Fig 6–21). This part of the test is positive if pain is created. The second part of the test is performed with the knee flexed and longitudinal compression applied with the knee in different altitudes of flexion. Pain produced with the knee flexed beyond 90 degrees indicates a posterior tear. If the pain occurs with the knee flexed less than 90 degrees, an anterior problem is suspected.

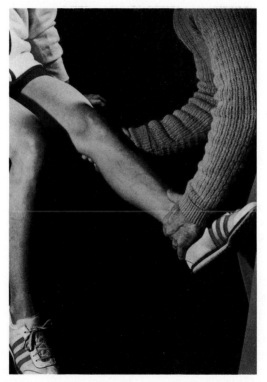

Fig 6–20.—To test the meniscus, grasp the ankle with the knee flexed, extend and externally rotate the knee. Pain or a click in the knee indicates a torn meniscus.

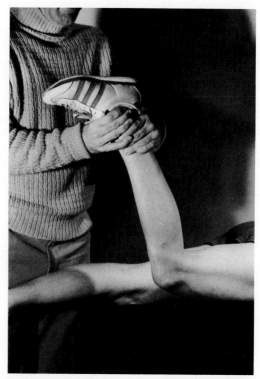

Fig 6–21. — To differentiate a torn meniscus from a ligament injury, Apley's test is performed. Lifting the prone leg from the examining table and applying torque to the knee will elicit pain in a ligament injury, but not in a meniscal injury.

Occasionally an athlete with normal knees complains of knee pain. Pathology in the hip and occasionally in the back can refer pain to the knee and must be considered.

Hamstring Pull

The hamstrings are subject to injury in any sport that involves running. Long-distance runners whose hamstrings become overdeveloped are particularly susceptible. A maximal effort or stepping wrong during the course of a workout causes an acute or gradual onset of pain in the medial or lateral thigh. The patient is unable to run without pain. Often he has an antalgic gait when running. In severe cases, walking is painful. Examination usually reveals a localized area of tenderness. If the pull has occurred several days before, there may be some discoloration in the thigh area. X-rays are not helpful.

Initially the treatment is application of ice and restriction of activities. After 72 hours, heat is begun. Salicylates, used as an anti-inflammatory agent, may be helpful. Return to full activities will take many weeks to many months, and the athlete will usually get impatient. However, premature return will produce further damage leading to chronicity. As the localized tenderness and pain subside, gradual stretching exercises can be instituted.

Quadriceps Rupture

A sudden sustained effort or direct blow may cause rupture of all or a portion of the quadriceps mechanism. The athlete complains of sudden pain followed by swelling in the thigh. Examination may reveal a palpable defect. There may be obvious weakness of knee extension. If the injury is more than several hours old there is usually so much swelling that an accurate diagnosis cannot be made. After the swelling subsides, the muscle may appear as a rolled-up mass in the anterior thigh. X-rays should be obtained but are usually normal.

If the injury is seen early, surgical treatment is indicated. If the patient is seen late or the diagnosis is made late, after the swelling has gone down, the athlete should be assured that the tenderness will gradually decrease. The muscle will function normally except when under maximum stress; then soreness may return. However, there will always be the cosmetic defect of the rolled-up muscle, which is usually insignificant. It may be 6–8 weeks before the athlete can return to activity.

Knee Problems

Unstable Knee

The athlete with an unstable knee complains of it giving way. There is a lack of trust when the knee bears weight, particularly on stairs or on uneven ground. The unstable knee is caused by an injury to the ligaments and/or joint capsule, a tear of the anterior or posterior cruciate or a partial tear of a collateral ligament associated with a capsular tear. Examination of the knee should include testing the medial and lateral collateral ligaments, the cruciate ligaments, and a McMurray's test, all previously described. A subtle tear of the meniscus, particularly in the posterior portion, may be the cause of instability. Differentiation of the problem is often so obscure that only the most experienced physician can achieve it.

Treatment of instability problems should be in the hands of the most experienced. Therefore, referral to a sports-oriented orthopedist should be made.

Chondromalacia of the Patella

Chondromalacia of the patella is not well understood. There are several theories of its cause. One is that it is precipitated by a single episode of trauma, such as falling on the flexed knee. It may be caused by multiple episodes of small trauma. In some instances it is caused by an abnormally lateral attachment of the patellar tendon, creating a displaced patella with flexion. This places the patella more in contact with the femoral condyle. Finally, there may be a genetic predisposition, with some individuals having a less resilient cartilage covering on all joints. Whatever the cause, the athlete complains of vague pain within the knee that may be localized behind the patella. There may be some swelling and increased discomfort going up and down stairs. Running on hills increases the pain.

Physical examination often reveals mild quadriceps atrophy. There may be no swelling. Tests of the cruciates and collateral ligaments and the menisci are normal. There may be lateral displacement of the insertion of the patellar tendon, an increased Q angle (see p. 124). The knee should be fully extended, the patella displaced distally with the examining hand and the patient asked to tighten the quadriceps mechanism. This may reproduce pain and/or grating, Palpation of the under surface of the patella may cause pain, particularly on the medial facet.

With increased interest in distance running, more knee problems are being seen. As an athlete increases his distance

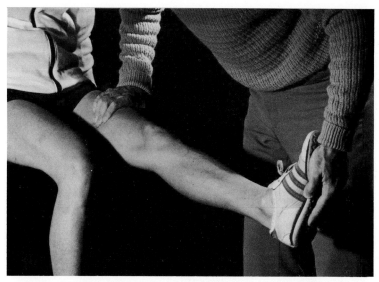

Fig 6–22. — The tightness or contracture in the Achilles tendon is checked by comparing dorsiflexion of the foot with the knee extended and with the knee flexed. This differentiates gastrocnemius from soleus contracture.

his posterior muscles, particularly the Achilles tendon muscles, become overdeveloped and shortened. This may cause abnormal stresses about the knee, exacerbating chondromalacia. Tightness of the postaxial muscles in the lower extremities should be checked (Fig 6–22). Routine x-rays of the knee are usually normal. Skyline views of the patella may reveal shallowness of the lateral femoral condyle.

Treatment of chondromalacia can be difficult. If at all possible, the physician should determine the exact cause, i.e., trauma, an anatomical malalignment, muscle tightness or a nonspecific cause. Stopping or at least altering the activity that has produced the problem or using a splint will help to relieve discomfort. Anti-inflammatory agents occasionally are helpful. There is evidence from the literature that aspirin has a regenerating effect on articular cartilage. The author has obtained good relief in many patients by prescribing 2 aspirin after each meal for 6–12 weeks.

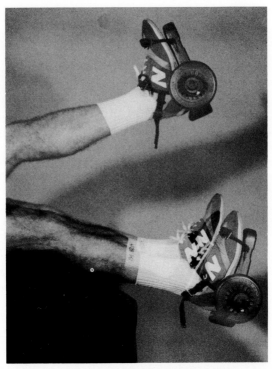

Fig 6–23.—Straight-leg raising with weights helps to strengthen the knee in athletes with chondromalacia and tendinitis about the knee.

Quadriceps-strengthening exercises also help. They should be done with the knee extended, first without weight and then with the addition of weights (Fig 6–23). Often the vastus medialis portion of the quadriceps mechanism is underdeveloped, and prescribing vastus medialis-squeezing exercises may help to stabilize the patella. This exercise is done by placing either a rolled towel or the athlete's fist between the knees and squeezing the knees together while at the same time internally rotating the leg. This position is held for 10 seconds. Multiple repetitions will gradually strengthen this portion of the quadriceps mechanism. In more advanced problems none of these treatments will be helpful. Surgery may be necessary if the athlete is going to continue to participate in sports.

Patellar Tendinitis (Runner's Knee, Jumper's Knee)

Inflammation of the patellar tendon at its attachment to the inferior pole of the patella (Fig 6–24) will create problems in the athlete who runs or jumps. The athlete will complain of pain as he pushes off, as in jumping. The runner will complain of pain after running for a period of time. There is usually no swelling. The athlete should be questioned as to how much time he spends stretching and warming up. Examination usually reveals tenderness only at the inferior pole of the patella. In long-distance runners there is usually tightness of the Achilles tendon group and the hamstring group.

Rest is the most effective treatment and should be continued until the symptoms are gone. Quadriceps-strengthening exercises in the straight-leg position should be done during the rehabilitation period. Long-distance runners should be encouraged to stretch the hamstring and Achilles tendon group. Occasionally this problem can be precipitated by abnormal foot plant, which may not be evident until the tight muscles have been stretched and the quadriceps has been

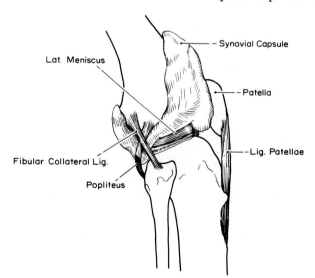

Fig 6–24.—The patellar tendon may become inflamed at the attachments on either the patella or the tibia.

strengthened. If the condition persists or recurs an orthotic device, such as an arch support, may cure the problem.

Bursitis of the Knee

There are many bursa around the knee (Fig 6–25), all of which are prone to inflammation, either following direct trauma or through overuse. The bursa become swollen to protect contiguous moving parts. The athlete complains of pain in one of the areas of the bursa. Examination reveals localized tenderness and, usually, swelling. X-rays are not helpful.

Often restriction of motion and warm compresses will largely alleviate the symptoms. So will aspirin taken as an anti-inflammatory agent. Occasionally, one of the stronger anti-inflammatory agents may be necessary. In the chronic case or in a well-localized acute problem, an injection of corticosteroid will prove effective. Occasionally, a chronic bursa will need to be surgically removed.

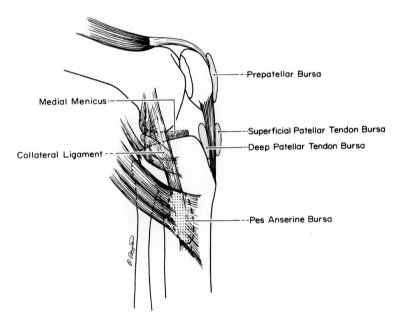

Fig 6–25. — The major problem bursae around the knee and their relationship to the tendons, ligaments and cartilage.

Baker's Cyst

Swelling in the popliteal area, either nondescript or well delineated, may indicate a Baker's cyst, the diagnosis applied to a mass in this region whether it be caused by bursitis of the semimembranous or the medial gastrocnemius. It also may be a result of a synovial hernia or a defect of the medial meniscus. The athlete complains of a full feeling in the popliteal area, particularly on extension of the knee. The mass may be palpable, and it may vary in size on any given day. Examination is best carried out by viewing the athlete from behind with the knee hyperextended. The cyst may be visible. Palpation of the popliteal area will reveal a lesion that feels like a cyst. Routine x-rays are usually normal, unless there is some preexisting degenerative arthritis. Fluid produced in the knee from arthritis may cause a synovial hernia. It is often wise to get an arthrogram, which can delineate the extent of the cyst. The cyst may extend down into the calf.

If the cyst is not causing any problems, no active treatment is necessary. However, if there is discomfort or limitation of function, surgical excision should be considered; but surgery should not be done until the etiology has been determined, if possible.

Recurrent Dislocation of the Patella

Recurrent dislocation of the patella is more common in girls than in boys. Several factors may predispose to recurrent dislocation. Patellar alta, or high-riding patella, is thought to be one. The patella is not well seated in the intertrabecular groove and has a greater likelihood of displacing laterally. Underdevelopment of the lateral femoral condyle allows the patella to dislocate laterally. Genu valgum, in which the quadriceps tendon is more lateral, predisposes to dislocations. This is particularly true in women, with the wide pelvis causing the femur to be internally angulated and placing the knee in a relative valgus position. A final factor is an increased Q angle (see p. 124). Lateral subluxation or dislocation is more likely. Examination reveals one or more of these conditions. Usually there is some subpatellar crepitus, indicating roughness of the patellar cartilage. The patella usually dislocates when the knee is flexed. The athlete may resist attempts to dislocate the patella because it is uncomfortable.

Vigorous physical therapy should be instituted to strengthen the quadriceps mechanism, especially the vastus medialis. If the patella continues to dislocate, surgery to realign the extensor mechanism is necessary.

Pellegrini Stieda Disease

Injury to the medial collateral ligament, producing either a partial tear or a hematoma, may lead to calcification within that area. It is most frequently found in the proximal portion of the medial collateral ligament attachment on the femur. The athlete complains of soreness and discomfort in this area with strenuous activity. There may be some swelling. X-rays show calcified densities in the region immediately adjacent to the femur, below the adductor tubercle.

Vigorous exercise and quadriceps strengthening often re-

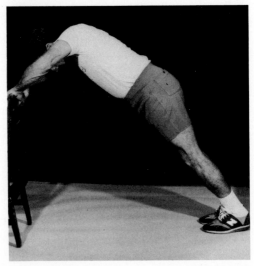

Fig 6–26.—The Achilles tendon is stretched by leaning forward with the feet on the floor and the knees and hips extended until stress is felt in the tendon. This position is held for 20 sec, and the exercise is repeated for 3–5 min.

lieve most of the symptoms. Occasionally, an injection of steroids may help relieve the pain. Surgery is rarely necessary.

Knee Pain in Runners

With the advent of interest in long-distance running, many athletes have complaints of knee pain. The runner usually experiences onset of pain after several miles. The knee becomes progressively more painful, so that running is no longer possible. A short time of walking will usually relieve the symptoms so that running may be resumed for a short distance, only to have the pain recur. Common areas of pain are the medial joint line and the lateral joint line. Careful questioning usually elicits the fact that an abnormally long distance has been run recently or that the runner's training has increased rapidly. Examination reveals no knee abnormali-

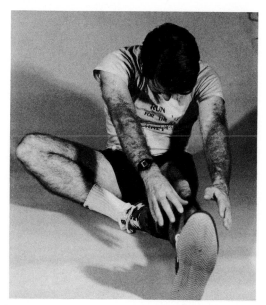

Fig 6–27.—The hamstrings are stretched by sitting in the position shown, trying to touch the nose to the knee and holding that position for 20 sec. The exercise is repeated for 3–5 min.

ties. However, examination of the foot and ankle usually reveals loss of flexibility of the Achilles tendon. The runner will not be able to dorsiflex the foot beyond neutral with the knee extended. In runners who complain of medial knee pain, the configuration of a normal or cavus arch combined with slight valgus of the knee is often seen. In runners with lateral knee pain, just the opposite, or a planus foot with genu varum, is common.

The athlete's running program must be curtailed but need not be stopped. An intensive stretching program focusing on stretching the Achilles tendon and the hamstrings is necessary. It is also helpful to strengthen the anterior tibial muscles (Figs 6–26 to 6–28). Frequently this is all that is necessary. A more rapid response to the pain syndrome, however, may be achieved by using an orthotic device in the running shoe.

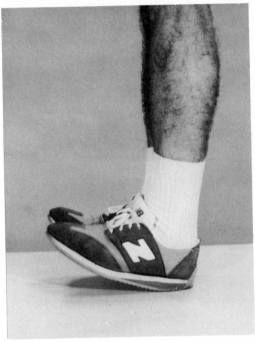

Fig 6–28.—Toe rises to strengthen the anterior tibial muscle and stretch the Achilles tendon.

Leg and Ankle Problems

Achilles Tendinitis

Pain at the Achilles tendon attachment to the os calcis is a common problem in runners. The athlete complains that aching starts in the area of the Achilles tendon after he runs a short distance. The same complaint is seen in tennis players. Often the athlete has tried a period of rest, only to have the pain recur. Examination reveals tenderness in the region of the Achilles tendon at the insertion on the os calcis or in the midportion of the tendon or at the musculotendinous junction about 3 inches from the os calcis. There may be crepitus that can be felt along the course of the tendon. There may be thickening and nodularity of the tendon. Examination of the range of motion of the ankle will demonstrate restricted dorsiflexion with the knee extended, produced by a tightness of the Achilles tendon group. X-rays should be obtained. In the longstanding problem, there may be calcium deposits within the substance of the tendon.

Continuing to participate in athletic endeavors with the tendon inflamed invites the risk of complete rupture of the tendon. The athlete must rest and elevate the heel. Frequently the symptoms are so severe that casting is necessary to completely rest the ankle joint. Anti-inflammatory agents, salicylates first, should be tried. Injection of the tendon sheath with steroids is not advised. If rest reduces the symptomatology, stretching of the Achilles tendon group and strengthening of the anterior muscles are begun. Running should not be allowed until the soreness has completely abated and the tendon is normal. If calcium has been shown on x-ray, conservative treatment is usually unsuccessful. Surgery is necessary unless the athlete wants to restrict his activities permanently.

Rupture of the Plantaris (Tennis Leg)

Sudden onset of pain in the calf while playing a racket sport or while running usually signifies rupture of the plantaris tendon. This is a small muscle located in the gastro-soleus group with a very small, pencil-like tendon, which inserts medially on the os calcis. The athlete complains of planting the foot to make a turn and the onset of a sharp pain, which feels as if "a golf ball hit me in the leg." Pain and inability to run ensue. This is a common injury in athletes over 30 years of age. It frequently occurs early in the season before the legs are in good shape. Examination reveals a tender area in the midportion of the body of the gastro-soleus muscle group, and occasionally some discoloration. X-rays are not indicated.

Reassurance is all the treatment that is needed. Local application of ice in the acute stages followed by heat after 72 hours usually takes care of the majority of the symptoms. Placing an elevation in the heel will relieve the stress on the tender area. The problem is self-limiting and requires about 6 weeks for full resolution. Activities may be resumed as the athlete feels comfortable.

Shin Splints

Pain along the anterior medial or lateral surface of the tibia in the early part of the training season is termed shin splints. It is thought that it is a periostitis of the attachment of the anterior tibial or the posterior tibial muscles along the border of the tibia. The athlete complains that the shin area becomes very painful. Occasionally there are complaints of swelling. Examination reveals tender areas along the anterior lateral aspect of the tibia or the anterior medial aspect, normally the midportion.

Resting the injured area will usually effect a cure. Strapping the ankles will reduce stress on the anterior or the posterior tibial muscles. In many instances there is tightness of the Achilles tendon group. Stretching of that group coupled with strengthening through isometric contractions of the anterior or posterior tibial muscles will gradually help the condition. The athlete should be counseled on the necessity for adequate warm-up and cool-down periods. Occasionally the problem can be created by excessive pronation of the foot, when an orthotic device will be necessary to prevent recurrence.

Peroneal Tendinitis

Inflammation of the peroneal tendon can occur from excessive eversion activity, a single incident or a series of repeated incidents. Continuing to run in worn-down shoes is often a

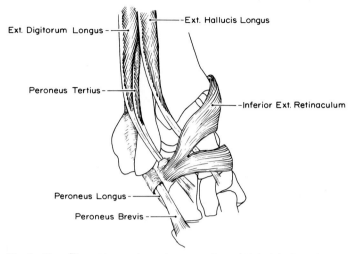

Ext. Digitorum Longus

Ext. Hallucis Longus

Peroneus Tertius

Inferior Ext. Retinaculum

Peroneus Longus

Peroneus Brevis

Fig 6–29. — The peroneal tendons are located behind and around the lateral malleolus.

predisposing factor. The athlete complains of pain over the lateral border of the foot and ankle (Fig 6 – 29). If he complains of a feeling that something is slipping out of place, subluxation should be suspected. A previous ankle sprain is usually part of the history. Examination reveals tenderness along the peroneal tendon, particularly at the insertion of the base of the fifth metatarsal. Resistance to eversion of the foot re-creates the pain.

In the case of tendinitis without subluxation, rest of the extremity will usually produce cure. The tendon can be protected to some extent during normal walking by putting an elevation along the lateral border of the foot inside the shoe. Anti-inflammatory agents may also assist. If a subluxing peroneal tendon is suspected, surgery is necessary.

Contusion Peroneal Nerve (Foot Drop)

The peroneal nerve passes behind the head of the fibula, near the skin surface. In this position, it is frequently injured by direct blows, which cause numbness and tingling in the nerve's distribution. If there is significant swelling or hemorrhage into the nerve sheath, there may be loss of motor function. Examination reveals decreased or absent sensation over the lateral leg. The athlete will not be able to dorsiflex his foot with significant strength. X-rays should be obtained to rule out a fracture of the fibular head.

Recovery is usually spontaneous. The initial swelling should be treated with ice for several days, followed by heat. In the case of a foot drop, the foot should be supported with a cast, brace or splint. The more rapid the return of sensory function the more favorable the prognosis. Fortunately, most athletes recover full function. There are few indications for surgery. Exquisite continuing pain may indicate intraneural scarring. A period of little or no nerve dysfunction followed in several weeks by gradually increasing paresthesias in the distribution of the peroneal nerve and weakness of dorsiflexion may indicate scarring. In these instances, surgical exploration of the nerve is indicated. During recovery, exercises to strengthen the dorsiflexors and the intrinsic muscles should be given. Peroneal strengthening exercises can be either isotonic or isometric. Strengthening of the intrinsic muscles of the foot can be done by ground-gripping toe exercise or by picking up marbles with the toes.

Ankle Sprain

As discussed in Chapter 7, sprain of the ankle is one of the most common injuries in all of athletics. The patient seen in the office is usually one in whom tenderness and swelling has persisted beyond a week or two. This ankle problem is most likely a second-degree injury with a partial ligament tear. A first-degree injury will usually be well by that time. A third-degree injury will show instability. Examination will reveal swelling and tenderness over the particular ligament that has been injured. The ankle joint should be tested for stability. X-rays should be obtained, but are usually negative.

In some instances no treatment, only reassurance, is all that is needed. Depending on the severity of the symptoms, taping of the ankle may be necessary. With the most severe symptoms, a short leg cast is indicated. Normally the physician will not go wrong by immobilizing the ankle for 10–14 days, after which the patient should be examined again. After removal of the cast, strengthening exercises of the anterior and posterior tibial muscles, the peroneal muscles and the gastro-soleus muscles should be started.

Stress Fractures about the Ankle

Stress fractures about the ankle are the second most common location for breaks. (Metatarsal stress fractures are the most common.) The most frequent location is the shaft of the fibula, about an inch and a half proximal to the tip. Occasionally an athlete with marked tibial torsion and genu varum will have a stress fracture of the tibia in the same location. Stress fractures can be confused with shin splints, Achilles tendinitis, peroneal tendinitis or chronic ankle sprain. The athlete complains of a gradual onset of pain. Examination is often unremarkable. In the more advanced stress fracture, some periosteal thickening and tenderness may be found. X-rays taken within the first 2 or 3 weeks may be normal. If the athlete continues to complain of pain, x-rays should be repeated 7–14 days later. Normally, by 6 weeks the x-rays will be positive.

Once the diagnosis is made, athletic activity must be stopped until the symptoms have cleared. It is usually not necessary to apply a cast. Two reasons for a cast are to be sure that the athlete rests the extremity and to assure patient comfort. It may take 10–12 weeks for the fracture to heal.

Foot Problems

Bursitis

The bursa anterior to the Achilles tendon at the heel or the one in the region of the attachment of the Achilles tendon to the os calcis can become inflamed. The athlete complains of pain in that area. Frequently there is swelling. Examination reveals tenderness in the heel distal or anterior to the insertion of the Achilles tendon, depending on which bursa is inflamed. There may be a fluctuant mass, indicating fluid within the bursal space. X-rays usually are normal, except for soft tissue swelling.

Friction over the bony prominence of the os calcis is frequently caused by poorly fitting shoes or a too-tight heel counter. New shoes or a softer heel counter may be necessary. Often the discomfort can be relieved by a piece of felt padding proximal to the tender area. If these simple measures do not work, steroid injections may be helpful. Rarely is surgery necessary.

Plantar Fasciitis (Heel Spur)

Inflammation of the plantar fascia causes complaints of pain in the posterior aspect of the heel where the plantar ligament attaches to the calcaneous (Fig 6–30). The athlete first complains that it is painful to run. As the problem gets worse, even walking becomes uncomfortable. A frequent complaint is heel pain after getting out of bed, which clears after 20–30 steps. Examination reveals local tenderness at the point of insertion of the plantar ligament on the os calcis. An antalgic gait is evident in the more severe cases. X-rays are usually normal, but in the athlete with long-standing complaints a forward projecting spur may be present (Fig 6–31).

Protecting the painful area is important. This can be accomplished by placing a felt pad with a cutout over the tender area or by using a plastic heel cup to absorb the shock of activity. In long-distance runners it is particularly important to examine the tension in the Achilles tendon, which is usually tight. Often a cure cannot be obtained unless the Achilles tendon muscle group is made more flexible. An arch support is sometimes

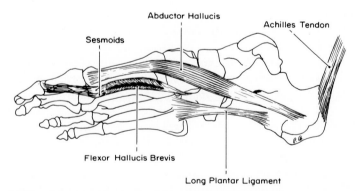

Fig 6–30.—The long plantar ligament attaches to the os calcis proximally and to the metatarsal area distally.

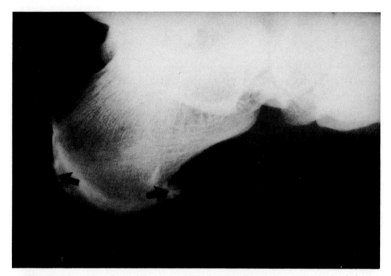

Fig 6–31. — X-ray of the os calcis, showing a spur on the plantar aspect at the attachment of the long plantar ligament. There is also a spur at the attachment of the Achilles tendon.

helpful. An injection of cortisone into the tender area may be necessary. In resistant cases, removal of the spur and stripping of the plantar fascia may be the only recourse. This is rarely required.

Metatarsalgia

Pain in the front portion of the foot can be caused by collapse of the transverse arch. The pain may be described as a dull ache or it may be a cramp. Examination often reveals a broadened forefoot. There may be localized tenderness underneath the metatarsal head area and mild to moderate deformity of the toes, indicating some intrinsic muscle imbalance. If the patient is asked to push the toes into the floor, he may be unable to lift the metatarsal heads from the surface, again indicating intrinsic weakness.

Exercises for the intrinsic muscles of the toes are often helpful. Have the patient consciously try to grip the floor with the toes as he walks. Another method is to have the athlete pick up

marbles with his toes. Frequently, while the patient under-
goes this rehabilitation program, supporting the foot with an
arch device is helpful. Obtaining a cure is often slow.

Morton's Foot

Pain in the forefoot is often attributed to an anatomical variance called Morton's foot. In this problem the second metatarsal is significantly longer than the first, creating a weight-dis-
tribution problem. For instance, if the weight-bearing in the
forefoot is divided into 6 equal parts, the normal foot will have
2 parts on the first metatarsal and 1 on each of the other 4 metatarsals. With a long second metatarsal, more weight is concen-
trated in that area than on the first. This causes thickening of
the second metatarsal shaft and may cause some displacement
of the sesamoids. A thick callus often develops beneath the
second metatarsal head. In the mechanics of running, as the
weight-bearing is progressively transmitted to the medial aspect of the foot, the shortened first metatarsal creates a functional mechanical problem manifested by forefoot pain. Examination reveals a thickened callus underneath the second
metatarsal, which is often tender. The second toe is noticeably
longer than the first. X-rays show that the increased length is
due to a longer metatarsal, rather than to an increased phalangeal length. The second metatarsal shows cortical thickening.

The main complaint is usually tenderness underneath the
second metatarsal head. Placing a metatarsal pad behind the
region of the callus will often relieve the symptoms and gradually decrease the thickness of the callus. For a long-term cure,
it is usually best to provide an orthotic device to support the
shortened first metatarsal, as well as to place the pressure of
weight-bearing on the second metatarsal proximally.

Morton's Neuroma

Irritation of the plantar digital nerve between the third and
fourth toes is a common problem in women, but it may occur
in men. The athlete complains of a sharp pain radiating into
the third and fourth toes without sharp delineation of its origin
(Fig 6–32). The pain usually develops after activity has been
going on for a time. Symptoms may be relieved by removing
the shoe and manually manipulating the lateral aspect of the

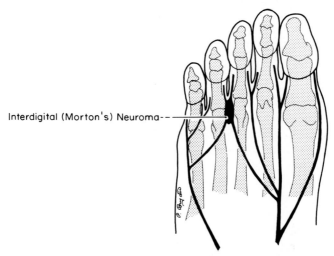

Interdigital (Morton's) Neuroma--

Fig 6–32. — Morton's interdigital neuroma usually occurs between the 3d and 4th metatarsals. This 2d metatarsal is also slightly long, indicating Morton's foot.

foot. As the problem progresses, the frequency of attacks increases. There may be pain radiating proximally toward the ankle joint. Examination reveals tenderness between the third and fourth toes. Occasionally a small nodule may be palpated. Rarely is there sensory loss in the distribution of the interdigital nerve. X-rays are usually normal.

Conservative treatment—applying a pad to help widen the intermetatarsal area during weight-bearing—should be tried but is usually not successful. Injecting the neuromal area with steroids often provides temporary relief. In those patients who do not respond to conservative treatment, surgical excision of the neuroma is indicated.

Foot Strain

The term "foot strain" denotes injury to the ligaments of the arch of the foot. The muscles of the foot that help support the bony arches in a dynamic way are functionally inadequate, either because of loss of strength or malpositioning. The stress of weight-bearing falls on the tarsal ligaments. This problem usually arises in those athletes with pes planus or pronated foot, more commonly called flat foot. Excessive training in the standing position, either walking or running, causes the athlete to complain of pain along the midborder of the foot, usually in the direction of the longitudinal arch. Occasionally there are complaints of calf pain. Examination usually reveals a pronated foot with frequent tenderness along the midportion of the arch of the foot but no swelling. X-rays, other than showing a flat foot, are usually normal. Occasionally, some athletes with a cavus or high-arch foot will complain of similar pain. In these instances, the cause of the pain is loss of foot flexibility. More often, the pain is located more laterally.

Foot strain associated with pes planus should be treated with exercises to strengthen the calf and foot muscles. Dorsiflexors, plantar flexors, evertors and invertors should all be conditioned. In addition, the intrinsic muscles of the foot should be exercised as described on page 145. If exercises are not successful, support with an orthotic device may give relief. For the athlete with a cavus foot, exercises are not particularly rewarding and a soft orthotic device is generally needed.

Stress Fracture

Stress fractures are produced by too much activity too soon or by too much activity all at once. The athlete often has run or hiked more or farther than usual. There is an onset of a vague ache in the midportion of the foot which becomes painful with continued activity. Examination usually reveals tenderness in the region of the second or third metatarsal shaft, and occasional swelling. If the symptoms have been present for several weeks, thickening of the metatarsal cortex may be palpable. X-rays, if taken prior to 10–21 days, may be normal. Repeat x-rays will demonstrate either early callus formation or periosteal thickening, if not a linear crack.

The fracture will heal spontaneously if stress is removed. Symptoms can be relieved by a metatarsal pad, heat and a mild analgesic. Occasionally in severe cases, a short leg cast will make the athlete more comfortable. It will usually take 3–4 weeks for the fracture to heal, and occasionally as long as 6 weeks.

Freiberg's Disease

Freiberg's disease should be suspected when an athlete complains of pain underneath the second metatarsal head. It normally occurs in the younger athlete. Examination reveals tenderness over the second metatarsal head, with or without thickening of the skin. Movements of the second metatarsal phalangeal joint are usually painful and restricted. X-rays of the foot show an abnormal-looking second metatarsal head, usually flattened and perhaps more sclerotic.

Rest may reduce the symptomatology and allow the metatarsal head to heal. If the problem is seen late, placing the weight-bearing more proximally on the metatarsal shaft by using a metatarsal pad will often relieve the symptoms. In refractory cases, excision of the metatarsal head is indicated. If this is necessary, the athlete needs to be reminded that it will shift excessive weight onto the third metatarsal head and may cause callus formation. In that instance, a metatarsal pad or arch support will be necessary. Therefore, in the initial treatment an arch support should be tried before surgery.

Sesamoiditis

Pain beneath the second metatarsal head can be due to a problem with the medial or lateral sesamoid (see Fig 6–28). There may be a history of landing on the ball of the foot. Occasionally a cleat, such as in soccer or baseball, underneath the ball of the foot can create enough irritation to produce problems in articulation between the sesamoid and the first metatarsal head. The athlete complains of pain in the ball of the foot, especially in running activities that involve sprinting. Examination reveals tenderness beneath the first metatarsal head which may be localized enough to be attributed to either the medial or the lateral sesamoid. The examiner flexes the toe and traps the sesamoids by applying pressure directly over the proximal portion of the metatarsal head. Extending the toe reproduces the symptoms. X-rays should be obtained to determine if the sesamoid is fractured. Sesamoids, however, are frequently in two parts. If there is any question of a fracture versus a bipartite sesamoid, the other toe should be x-rayed.

Special skyline views can be obtained to delineate the articular surface.

If x-rays show a fracture, the foot should be immobilized in a cast for several weeks. If there is no fracture, resting the area by placing a pad next to the metatarsal head and restricting activity will allow symptoms to abate. In some instances, injection of the first metatarsal joint with a small amount of cortisone will reduce the symptoms. If symptoms persist, consideration can be given to removing the sesamoid. However, this should be considered with caution.

Hammer Toe

Hammer toe is caused by a fixed flexion deformity of the interphalangeal joint. The etiology of the deformity is unclear, but it is probably due to a primary muscle imbalance or to an imbalance secondary to a nerve problem. The athlete usually complains of pain in the toes on the plantar aspect of the tips. There is usually a painful, thick callus over the dorsal aspect of the proximal interphalangeal (PIP) joint. X-rays demonstrate flexion of the PIP joint and either flexion or extension of the distal interphalangeal joint.

If symptoms are mild and the flexion deformity of the PIP joint is not too acute, putting a metatarsal bar or pad in the shoe elevates the metatarsal head. This creates some extension of the joint, relieving the symptoms. In more severe cases, surgery to straighten the toe relieves the pain and callus.

Bunions and Hallus Valgus

Bunions are more common in women but are occasionally seen in men. Though the problem is more frequent in the older women, it can still be seen in teenagers and young adults. The athlete complains of pain, swelling and occasionally redness over the first metatarsal phalangeal joint. Examination reveals prominence over the first metatarsal head with overlying swelling. In the acute phases, the swollen area will be tender and red. The great toe drifts laterally, creating a valgus position. X-rays usually show prominence of the first metatarsal head with an exostosis in that area. There is a hallux valgus.

The athlete with a mild hallux valgus requires no treatment but should be careful to wear shoes of the proper width. In moderate cases, relief of the symptoms over the first metatarsal head can be obtained by appropriate padding. Pads should be placed proximal to the metatarsal head so that friction is created between the felt padding and the shoes rather than the metatarsal head. In severe cases, surgery is necessary if the athlete is going to be comfortable enough to participate in sports.

Skin and Nail Problems

Blisters

Blisters are produced by excessive shearing forces between the skin and either the socks or the shoes. The outer layer of skin is gradually lifted away from the dermal layer and fills with fluid. If blood vessels are involved, the fluid may be tinged with blood. The safest treatment is to leave the blister intact. However, if it ruptures, the area should be cleansed well with soap and the entire bleb debrided. A clean, antibiotic-impregnated dressing can be applied for several days until the blister heals. Many athletes want their blisters opened because they think this allows them to get back to participation more quickly. There may be some validity in this. A blister to be ruptured should be cleansed thoroughly with soap. Using a small needle, make a hole at the base of the blister, express all fluid, and apply an antibiotic ointment. An alternate method would be to rupture the blister, remove the entire bleb and paint the area with an antiseptic solution. This is very uncomfortable; but if the antiseptic solution contains alcohol, the alcohol will deaden the nerve endings. After the initial discomfort, the blister will not be too sensitive. It should still be kept clean and dry.

Callosities

A callosity is a localized thickening of the dermis caused by abnormal pressures. Common areas for callosities are beneath the metatarsal heads, on the lateral border of the foot at the fifth metatarsal head, the medial border of foot at the first metatarsal head and along the medial border of the great toe.

Further inspection usually reveals either an abnormal bony prominence or some anatomical variance, such as a hammer toe or a bunion.

Treatment should be aimed at correcting the anatomical problem. If this is not feasible, the callus should be trimmed with a sharp blade or emery board to keep it thin in order to prevent pain. A callus can be kept soft with petrolatum, cocoa butter or hand lotion.

Corns

A corn is a very localized thickening of skin over a bony prominence, most frequently over the proximal interphalangeal joints of the toes, in the case of claw or hammer toes. Occasionally, corns are found between the toes, particularly the fourth and fifth, and occasionally the third and fourth.

Treatment initially should consist of trimming the corns carefully, except in athletes with diabetes. Corns may be padded to keep pressure away from the bony prominence. If this fails or is unacceptable, the corn should be excised and the bony prominence removed.

Ingrown Toenail

Infection along the medial or lateral border of the toenail is most frequently seen in the great toe. The cause is usually improper trimming of the toenail. The edge of the toenail gets beneath the medial or lateral pulp, creating a foreign-body reaction and subsequent inflammation. Examination usually reveals granular tissue on the corner of the nail and a surrounding cellulitis.

Treatment involves moving the edge of the nail back to the germinal matrix, which should be done using a local anesthetic. As the nail regrows, the paronychia should be kept away from the leading edge until it has grown beyond the pulp. This can be accomplished by keeping the area walled off with cotton.

Plantar Warts

Plantar warts, often confused with callosities, are similar to those found on any other area of the body. A wart is a papilloma growing out from the basal layers of the skin. These warts are usually symptomatic only if they are on the weight-bearing portion of the foot. Those on the heel and underneath the metatarsal heads cause the most problems. Examination reveals a calloused area with a slightly recessed, roughened papilloma in the center.

Treatment consists of trimming the wart to its base, which is then cauterized with liquid nitrogen, electrocautery or a chemical agent. Occasionally surgery is indicated.

Runner's Toe, Tennis Toe

Black toenails are a common complaint of many athletes, particularly runners and tennis players. The second toe is the most often affected, but the first and third may also have problems. The athlete complains that the toenail became black after activity. There may not be much pain associated with the problem. The subungual hematoma is produced by pressure on the nail by the end of the shoe or by a ridge in the shoe, causing minute elevation of the nail away from the nail bed. This produces hemorrhage, and gradually this space fills with blood.

For severe pain, it may be necessary to make a small hole in the nail to allow release of the subungual hematoma. If the pain is not severe, no treatment is indicated. The athlete should be warned that the nail may fall off, but a new one will grow underneath. The problem can recur if shoe fit is not corrected.

REHABILITATION

The physician's job is not complete until the athlete has returned to his previous level of competitive edge. The general goal is to return the athlete to the highest level of function in the shortest possible time. The physician should supervise this return to preinjury status, and the assistance of a physical therapist or athletic trainer may help to attain the goal. It is up to the physician to identify the particular functional area that is abnormal and develop a corrective program. A sound principle in achieving this goal is that the uninvolved extremity should be exercised in a manner similar to the injured one.

Once a program is started to restore a muscle to its previous functional level, there will be a certain period of soreness as the muscle is exercised. This can be minimized by a period of

5–7 days of breaking into the retraining regimen. Following this break-in period, the intensity of workouts can be increased. As in any other athletic endeavor, muscle-strengthening exercises should be preceded by warming up and stretching. Initially, the speed of movement should be moderate. Range of motion should be as great as possible within the limits of comfort. It must be remembered that full rehabilitation will only be regained when there is normal strength for the full range of motion. Initially, the amount of weight used must be heavy enough to require a maximum contraction. It is gauged by taking a particular weight, which the athlete thinks he can handle, and doing 8–10 repetitions. If at least 8 repetitions cannot be done, the weight is too great and should be decreased. Once the starting weight has been determined, more weight can be added at spaced intervals. As the athlete progresses in the rehabilitation program, a higher-intensity exercise period should be followed by a rest period of 24–48 hours.

Before the athlete is allowed to return to athletic competition, the injured area should be judged normal by the physician. Again, it is fortunate that there is the uninvolved opposite extremity available for comparison.

A WORD OF ADVICE

The physician treating exercise-related injuries will encounter athletes who emphasize that the professional athlete can recover from many conditions much more rapidly than has been indicated in these chapters. This is true, but professional athletes run a calculated risk, which most of them are prepared to take in order to continue functioning in their livelihood without missing a lot of "work time." In the exercise-related injury in the nonprofessional, the physician's duty should be to return the patient to that exercise as rapidly as possible, but consistent with thoughts of lifelong involvement in the activity.

SUGGESTED READING
General
1. Cozen, L.: *Office Orthopedics* (Springfield, Ill.: Charles C Thomas, Publisher, 1974).

2. Crenshaw, A. A.: *Campbell's Operative Orthopedics* (St. Louis, Mo.: C. V. Mosby Co., 1971).
3. *Measuring and Recording of Joint Motion* (Chicago: American Academy of Orthopedic Surgeons, 1965).
4. Salter, R. B.: *Textbook of Disorders and Injuries of the Musculoskeletal System* (Baltimore: Williams & Wilkins Co., 1970).

Shoulder
1. Bateman, J. E.: *The Shoulder and Environs* (St. Louis, Mo.: C. V. Mosby Co., 1965).
2. Moseley, H. F.: *Shoulder Lesions* (3d ed.; Baltimore, Williams & Wilkins Co., 1969).

Elbow
1. Smith, F. M.: *Surgery of the Elbow* (2d ed.; Philadelphia: W. B. Saunders Co., 1972).

Wrist
1. Linscheid, R. L., Dobyns, J. W., et al.: Traumatic instability of the wrist: Diagnosis, classification and pathomechanics, Bone Joint Surg. 54:1612, 1972.

Hand
1. Boyes, J., and Bunnell, S.: *Surgery of the Hand* (5th ed.; Philadelphia: J. B. Lippincott, 1970).

Spine
1. Rothman, R.: *Spine,* Vols. I and II (Philadelphia: W. B. Saunders Co., 1975).
2. Ruge, D., and Wilson, L.: *Spinal Disorders: Diagnosis and Treatment* (Philadelphia: W. B. Saunders Co., 1977).

Knee
1. Smillie, I. S.: *Injuries of the Knee Joint* (4th ed.; Baltimore, Williams & Wilkins Co., 1970).

Ankle
1. Bonnin, J. G.: *Injuries to the Ankle* (New York: Grune & Stratton, Inc., 1950).

Foot
1. Gianestras, N., et al.: *Foot Disorders: Medical and Surgical Management* (Philadelphia: Lea & Febiger, 1976).
2. Lewin, P.: *Foot and Ankle: Their Injuries, Disease, Deformities and Disabilities* (3d ed.; Philadelphia: Lea & Febiger, 1947).

Rehabilitation
1. Ryan, A. J., and Allman, F.: Rehabilitation of the Injured Athlete (Chap. 13) in *Sports Medicine* (New York: Academic Press, 1974).

7 / Evaluation of the Injured Athlete in the Arena

THE UNCONSCIOUS ATHLETE

The unconscious athlete presents a challenge. The physician knows that a head injury has occurred but has no way of knowing what other parts of the body may be injured. Until a complete examination can be obtained or until the athlete regains consciousness, every area of the body must be assumed to be injured. Injuries to the extremities are not particularly critical, but head and spinal injuries are.

The unconscious athlete should *not* be moved at all. An initial check should be made to be sure the airway is open. Vital signs should be obtained. The level of neurologic function should be delineated. Note should be taken whether the athlete, although unconscious, is moving any extremities. The size of the pupils and their reaction to light should be observed. Anatomical disalignment of all extremities should be noted. If the athlete is still unconscious after this cursory exam, under no circumstances should he be moved without stabilizing the spine, either on a board or with sandbags. The athlete should be carefully transferred to a backboard, maintaining traction on the neck to prevent any rotation, flexion or extension. The athlete should be constantly monitored as he is transported. This may require the physician to go with the patient in an ambulance to the closest emergency facility.

Many times, an athlete will be knocked unconscious for only a brief time. By the time the physician examines him, his head may be starting to clear. In these instances, it is often difficult to determine exactly what should be done. The level of consciousness and the athlete's memory of events must be checked. If the athlete can answer questions, has no spinal symptoms and can move his extremities, he can be moved from the arena without undue precautions. In general, if the player recovers in 2–3 minutes, if he can remember what has happened and if he has no abnormal vital signs, further examination can be delayed as long as observation continues. He should not be allowed to return to play. If, after 20–30 minutes of observation, there are no untoward sequelae and no tenderness in the cervical or thoracic region, then it may be safe to allow him to play.

Athletes with any other head injuries should be taken to the hospital for neurosurgical evaluation, which should include a thorough neurologic exam as well as x-rays of the skull and the spine. Athletes who have been unconscious for more than 5 minutes or who have amnesia should be observed in the hospital for 24–48 hours following complete neurosurgical evaluation. If an athlete complains of headaches following hospitalization, he should not be allowed to play until these have resolved and neurosurgical clearance has been given.

THE CONSCIOUS ATHLETE

Examining the conscious athlete in the arena should be done as quickly as possible. If the athlete is able to move all his extremities and has no spinal symptoms, it is safe to transport him from the playing area. Outside the field of action there is less stress on the player and on the physician, and a complete history can be obtained. The athlete should be allowed to describe in his own words exactly what happened, and any details that are left out should be specifically questioned. The location and the severity of the pain are important. Did the athlete feel any clicks or snaps or any instability at the time of injury? As much detail as possible should be recorded.

Which athletes should be allowed to return to play? Those who have transitory unconsciousness and who continue to be groggy for more than 2–3 minutes after injury should not play. The athlete who complains of tingling or numbness in his extremities should not play. If there is paraspinal tenderness or muscle guarding, play should not be allowed. Any player with an extremity injury that requires him to be carried from the field should not be allowed to return until a complete examination has been done.

A patient with an injured extremity should have clothes removed from it, and all taping and strapping taken off. Likewise, the opposite extremity should be completely bared. It is advantageous to examine the normal limb first for 2 reasons: (1), the physician can see what is normal for the individual athlete; (2), once the athlete has seen what the examination is going to be like, he is more likely to relax and allow a better examination of the injured area. If any anatomical malalignment exists, further examination should be done discreetly until proper x-rays can be obtained.

If the examination is done shortly after the injury, there may be no swelling. Swelling may indicate serious vessel damage. The extremity must be elevated with a compression dressing and the patient's vital signs checked frequently. The condition of the skin should be observed, as subtle bruising may be the only indication of the exact area of injury. When this general exam is complete, the specific examination of the injured part can begin.

GENERAL CONDITIONS

Contusions

Contusions are caused by a direct blow against the skin, which ruptures capillaries and fills the local area with blood. Damage may be limited to the subcutaneous tissue but often involves the muscle.

Treatment consists of elevating the extremity and applying ice for 12–24 hours. The extremity should be immobilized to encourage soft tissue healing and to prevent further injury. Gradual resumption of muscle function should be encouraged within the limits of pain.

Hematoma

Hematoma is a collection of blood in the soft tissues. Superficial hematoma is easy to diagnose, but blood within the muscle is more elusive. If it is not possible to make the diagnosis any other way, aspiration of the swelling should be attempted. If a hematoma is found, it should be evacuated as completely as possible. Some advocate the injection of an enzyme into the area to help control damage, but the author has not found this efficacious.

The limb should be elevated and immobilized to prevent further soft tissue injury. Ice and a compression dressing should be applied. Forty-eight to seventy-two hours following the injury, heat can be applied to increase the area's blood supply and aid resorption of the hemorrhage. The limb should be rested until swelling and soreness have dissipated. Active exercise can be started as soreness decreases. Specifically contraindicated in the treatment of hematomas is massage, because it often breaks up the clot and bleeding resumes. The result of this may be an increased incidence of myositis ossificans, a calcification in the soft tissues at the site of the hematoma.

Sprains

Sprains are probably the most common injury in all sports. The term "sprain" is often incorrectly interchanged with "strain." A sprain is an injury to a ligament, whereas a strain is an injury to a musculotendinous unit. Both injuries are graded in a similar manner, that is, according to the severity.

A *first-degree sprain* occurs when there has been stretching of the ligaments supporting a joint but no significant tearing of the soft tissue. Tenderness, swelling and stress pain are symptoms; there is often no effusion or hematoma, no pain on motion and no instability. Treatment includes rest for the injured joint — in the lower extremity, by the use of crutches and a soft wrap; in the upper extremity, by using a sling. A compression dressing can be applied during the first 24 – 48 hours to control hemorrhage. Some advocate using enzymes to help control the soft tissue reaction, but in our experience this has not proved beneficial. Once the swelling has subsided and the tenderness has decreased, usually 3 – 10 days after injury, early use of the injured part should be encouraged. Heat from whirlpool baths or tub soaks in water at 160 – 180 F is helpful.

In the late healing stages, contrast treatment may be utilized. This consists of packing the injured area in ice for 5 – 10 minutes, then removing the ice and applying heat. These treatments can be done for 20 – 30 minutes, 3 times a day. The patient should be able to use the extremity without discomfort in 7 – 10 days. This varies with the joint injured and the age of the patient. The more complex the motions of the joint, the longer the recovery period.

The *second-degree,* or moderate, *sprain* is often the most difficult to recognize and can be the most difficult to treat. In this injury there has been some tearing of the ligaments that help to stabilize the joint, but physical examination shows no such instability. If these partially torn ligaments are not supported, further injury may cause a third-degree sprain. Symptoms are pain, local tenderness, swelling, effusion and inability to use the joint.

Treatment involves rest, a compression dressing, cold packs and external support in the form of a rigid splint or a cast. Often, aspiration of the joint to remove the effusion makes the patient more comfortable. Again, the role of enzymes is questionable. The difficulty in treating this injury lies in determining the severity of the damage. A 10% tear of the ligament requires one period of immobilization, whereas a 90% tear necessitates longer immobilization. The physician must remember that treating a second-degree injury requires the same length of time as a fracture. Immobilization will generally be necessary for 3 weeks, after which time the joint should be re-examined to determine whether further support is necessary. It may be wise to decrease the amount of the immobilization by shifting from something rigid to something soft, such as a cast padding wrap or felt strapping. Gradually, immobilization is decreased over the next 7 – 14 days. When all external support has been removed, the joint should be mobilized with whirlpool baths, but the author has found that contrast baths, ice alternated with heat, as described previously, seem to be more effective.

The physician often will encounter problems in managing the patient with second-degree injuries. Problems arise after 3 weeks, when the swelling is down. The joint feels good, yet the physician knows that to return the athlete to activity only invites further trouble. A partially torn structure needs several weeks more to heal completely and to assure a functioning joint for future use.

Third-degree, or severe, *sprain* is indicated by joint instability. In this sprain, one or several ligaments that maintain joint stability have been completely disrupted. There is severe pain, blood within the joint, swelling, severe disability and abnormal motion. Often because of muscle guarding after the injury, instability may be missed. If all other symptoms are present and instability cannot be demonstrated, it may be necessary to anesthetize the joint to diagnose the instability. Occasionally, the instability will only be demonstrable by x-rays taken with the area under stress.

Treatment is often surgical for a third-degree knee sprain, but not always for an ankle sprain. It is probably best to refer any third-degree injury to a specialist for his judgment regarding operative and nonoperative management. If a nonoperative approach is chosen, the joint is immobilized in a plaster cast. X-rays are taken after casting to be sure the joint is aligned normally. Immobilization time varies with the joint, but it will be approximately the same as that required for a fractured bone.

Strains

A strain is an injury to a musculotendinous unit. Such injuries are classified like sprains: first-degree, second-degree and third-degree. A *first-degree,* or mild, *strain* occurs with stretching, but not tearing, of musculotendinous tissue. In the early stages, the tenderness is localized, but it becomes more generalized with time. There may or may not be swelling. Usually the problem will resolve itself in several days. The *second-degree strain* indicates more severe damage, with partial tearing of the musculotendinous unit. In addition to soreness, there is loss of strength, which may be minimal. The *third-degree strain,* a complete rupture of the musculotendinous unit, normally requires surgical repair if diagnosed early. Early diagnosis can be difficult because muscle spasms that start shortly after the injury can mask the signs.

The main treatment of first- and second-degree strains is protection from further injury, which requires several days' rest. This is especially important in treating second-degree strains. Splinting, taping or some other form of immoblization will be necessary, and the injured musculotendinous units must be mobilized slowly to prevent a chronic problem. Once chronicity has developed, it will take a long period of rest followed by a long period of rehabilitation to achieve a pain-free, strong muscle. The third-degree strain often requires surgery and should be treated by a specialist.

Dislocations

A dislocation is the loss of normal anatomical alignment of a joint. It is caused by the tearing of some tissues around the joint, creating a second- or third-degree sprain. Partial dislocation, called subluxation, is suspected when the patient complains of a feeling that the joint is slipping out when there is no true dislocation. Repeated injury to a subluxing joint may create a dislocation. Subluxation complaints should be thoroughly investigated and the muscular structures surrounding the joint rehabilitated.

After x-rays have delineated the extent of injury, a dislocation is treated by reduction. Because treatment often stops here, the results have not always been good. If the physician remembers that the dislocation has created a second- or third-degree injury to the joint, it is obvious that further treatment is necessary. A period of immobilization should follow reduction to allow torn tissue to heal. Specific dislocations will be discussed later in this chapter.

Fractures

A fracture is a loss of normal bone integrity. A simple fracture is one in which the bone is broken but the bone ends are not piercing the skin. A compound fracture is one in which the skin has been punctured by the broken bone. Both types of fractures are described as angulated, displaced, comminuted, or impacted. "Greenstick," or incomplete, fractures occur frequently in children and can be handled safely by most physicians. However, all other fractures should be referred to a qualified specialist for care.

The athlete, as well as his family and his coaches, need to know the time required for a fracture to heal. It takes approximately 3 weeks for a spiral fracture in a long bone to unite and

TABLE 7-1.—HEALING RATES OF
COMMON FRACTURES

BONE	TIME TO UNITE (WK)
Phalanges and metacarpals	3
Wrist	6
Radius and ulna	8
Humerus	3
Spine	12
Hip	12
Femur	12
Tibia and fibula	8
Ankle	6–8
Metatarsals phalanges	3
Navicular	16+
Os calcis	12+

6 weeks for firm consolidation. Transverse fractures and lower
limb fractures take 12 weeks. In children, these time requirements are halved. The healing rate will, of course, vary with
the patient's age, state of health, the degree of bone-end appo-
sition, the sufficiency of the blood supply and the effectiveness
of immobilization. Table 7–1 shows common fractures and
their usual healing rates.

REGIONAL ACUTE PROBLEMS

Head and Face

Lacerations

Lacerations occur frequently around the head and face and
usually bleed profusely, as the blood supply to this area is
very plentiful. A sterile dressing and compression should be
applied to control the hemorrhage until a more thorough examination can be done and treatment delineated. After necessary anesthesia has been administered, the wound should be
checked for injury to critical underlying structures, thoroughly
cleansed and any foreign bodies removed. When lacerations
involve muscle and tendinous structures, a specialist may
need to be consulted. If not, the subcutaneous tissue can be
approximated and the skin closed. Generally, scalp or facial
sutures can be removed in 5–7 days.

Nose

The nose is frequently injured and presents 2 problems: bleeding and airway obstruction. When the athlete is bleeding from the nose, he should be placed prone and an icebag applied to the area. If bleeding continues, the nose should be packed and ice applied. If the bleeding still does not stop, the athlete should be taken to a hospital for treatment. If the nasal bone or cartilage has been broken, there may be loss of normal anatomical configuration. Realignment and protection should be provided by an appropriate specialist.

Concussion

Concussion involves alteration in brain function following a blow to the head. There may be a brief loss of consciousness, a loss of memory for a few moments surrounding the injury, and/or mild visual disturbances and loss of normal equilibrium. These manifestations require further observation, and the athlete should not be allowed to return to play. If the symptoms do not clear in 5–10 minutes, the patient should be referred for complete neurological evaluation.

Neck Sprain and Torticollis

Injuries to the neck are produced by hyperflexion, hyperextension or rotatory stresses to the cervical region. The patient's main complaints are pain and limited motion. Physical findings include localized tenderness within the cervical region, possible muscle guarding and, most important, restricted motion. There is usually no neurological deficit. In the more severe injuries there may be tilting of the head to one side or the other—an acquired torticollis. If this is the case, an x-ray of the neck is necessary to rule out subluxation of the facet joints or fractures of the spinous or transverse processes.

Treatment consists of resting the neck; the patient should be confined to bed for 12–24 hours. A cervical collar may be necessary. Heat, massage and mild analgesics are helpful. Often the complaints will be mild immediately following the injury, but in 24–48 hours more severe symptoms will be present. If this is the case, muscle relaxants and traction may be added to the above regimen.

Contusion

Contusion of the neck region can occur either anteriorly or posteriorly. When bleeding occurs within the muscles, it is hard to differentiate from a sprain. Direct blows can create bone injury; thus, an x-ray should be obtained. If there is any indication of injury to the cervical spine, referral should be made to the appropriate specialist.

Treatment varies with the severity of injury. Usually ice, rest and an analgesic are all that are required. A cervical collar for several days will make the patient more comfortable. Activity may be resumed as soon as symptoms subside.

Thoracic and Lumbar Spine

Sprain

The thoracic and lumbar spine are frequent problem areas. The sprain most frequently occurs in those athletes who must apply maximum effort over a short period of time, such as a blocking football linemen or weight lifters. The athlete complains of general pain in either the upper or the lower back, where examination usually reveals an area of tenderness. Pain is caused by active muscle contraction or passive stretching of the injured area. There often may be muscle guarding on the side opposite the tender area as the paraspinal muscles attempt to restrict motion toward the injured side. In more severe injuries, there may be a muscular scoliosis of the spine. Neurological examination of the lower extremities should be performed; it will usually be normal. If there is any abnormality in the neurological exam, x-rays of the spine should probably be obtained.

Again, the best treatment is rest for the injured area. Local heat may help relieve the muscle guarding. Muscle relaxants are helpful. Mild to moderate analgesics may be required. As the pain begins to subside, the patient may be immobilized. Often some type of back support, either a strap or a corset, will speed mobilization. However, the athlete should not be returned to activity too soon, as this will only create a chronic condition. Once the symptoms begin to subside, an exercise program, using Williams or Regents exercises, will help rehabilitate the injured structures.

Shoulder and Arm

Fracture of the Clavicle

Fracture of the clavicle, more commonly seen in children than adults, occurs in the violent sports, usually from a direct blow. Because the clavicle is subcutaneous, it thus is more exposed for injury than other bones. A fracture may occur at either end but is most common in the middle portion. The patient complains of pain on motion; examination usually reveals obvious deformity and crepitus at the fracture site.

A figure 8 splint is used to immobilize the fracture for 3 weeks. In order for the immobilization to be effective, the shoulders must be pulled into hyperabduction, so that the patient looks much like a person standing at attention. Often, placing the corresponding arm in a sling for 2–3 days makes the patient more comfortable.

Fracture of the Humerus

Fracture of the humerus, either proximally at the surgical neck or distally in the shaft, occurs from direct blows or from having the arm caught in a compromised position in contact sports. Examination may not show any anatomical misalignment. In surgical neck fractures there is swelling, tenderness and painful motion, which may not be readily distinguishable from normal shoulder motion. In shaft fractures, there is tenderness and crepitus with false motion at the fracture site.

Fractures of the cervical neck are treated by immobilizing the arm in a sling for 3 weeks. Shoulder motion may resume about 10 days after injury. The patient is instructed to lean forward from the waist and swing the arm to and fro and in a circular motion. This activity helps to prevent the most frequent and serious complication of this fracture, a stiff shoulder.

Treatment of fractures of the humerus shaft can often be done with a sling also, but occasionally a hanging arm cast will be needed for traction. With both of these fractures, it is necessary for the patient to sleep sitting up for at least 3 weeks with the injured arm hanging free to maintain reduction and to increase comfort. Both these fractures are probably best treated by an orthopedist.

Dislocation of the Acromioclavicular Joint (Shoulder Separation)

Injury to the acromioclavicular joint is seen frequently in those sports where the athlete falls frequently. Falling on the outstretched arm with the elbow fully extended, falling directly on the point of the elbow with the elbow flexed or, occasionally, falling directly on the point of the shoulder creates a first-, second- or third-degree sprain of the acromioclavicular ligament. In the first-degree injury there may be nothing more than pain with some local tenderness. In the second-degree sprain there is usually pain, swelling and tenderness. Traction applied to the long axis of the arm will increase the discomfort. In the third-degree injury there probably is an anatomical step-off of the joint. If the acromioclavicular and coracoclavicular ligaments have been completely disrupted, the joint will be unstable. If there is any question regarding the diagnosis, stress views of the acromioclavicular joint should be obtained by taking an anterior view of the shoulder with the athlete holding a weight in his injured arm and comparing that view with one taken without the weight.

A first-degree sprain requires only simple immobilization in a sling for several days. Treatment of the second-degree injury requires immobilization in a Kenney-Howard sling to elevate the shoulder with maintenance of alignment by a cuff to provide compression over the acromioclavicular joint. The joint must be protected for 6 weeks. In a third-degree sprain, maintaining the reduction with a sling and a cuff is difficult because of the marked instability. The alternate treatment is an open reduction, using a pin or screw. Second- and third-degree injuries are probably best treated by the orthopedist.

Dislocation of the Shoulder

Dislocation of the glenohumeral, or shoulder, joint occurs when an athlete falls on the outstretched arm. These dislocations can occur anteriorly, posteriorly, or subglenoidly. The anterior dislocation is by far the most common. The athlete's immediate complaint is that he cannot use the arm. Inspection usually will reveal an anatomical deformity, frequently with the humeral head in front of the shoulder joint. Motion is pain-

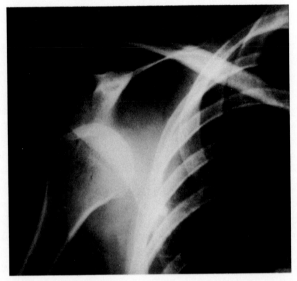

Fig 7–1. — Anterior inferior dislocation of the shoulder.

ful; internal rotation of the shoulder is impossible if the dislocation is anterior. In heavily muscled athletes, it is occasionally difficult to tell if the shoulder is dislocated. If there is any question, x-rays should be obtained for confirmation (Figs 7 – 1 and 7 – 2). Before any treatment, a neurologic examination of the upper extremity should be done, paying particular attention to the axillary nerve. The deltoid muscle is innervated by this nerve, but its function cannot be checked because of the discomfort associated with the injury. The same nerve supplies the sensation of the skin over the deltoid muscle; thus, checking that area will indicate the function of the nerve.

The dislocated shoulder should be reduced as soon as possible. It is absolutely necessary to have complete muscle relaxation for successful reduction. At the time of injury, before muscle guarding induced by pain has started, there is usually enough relaxation to reduce the dislocation. Any method that fixes the scapular position while applying traction to the humerus in the direction of the pull of muscle fibers will usually reduce the dislocation (Fig 7 – 3). If reduction cannot be easily

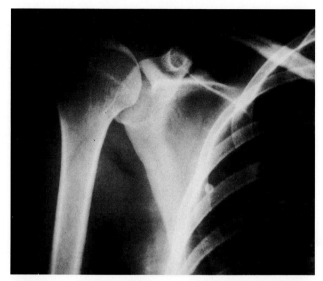

Fig 7–2. — Postreduction dislocation of the shoulder.

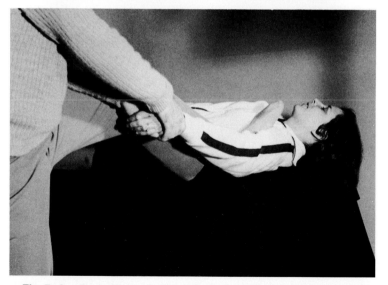

Fig 7–3. — Reduction of dislocated shoulder by applying gentle traction on the arm and using the foot in the axilla to apply counter-traction.

accomplished at the time of injury, the athlete should be taken to a hospital and x-rays obtained to document the type of dislocation. Administration of an analgesic and a muscle relaxant may then provide enough relaxation. Post-reduction x-rays should always be obtained. The injured arm should be immobilized in the sling for 3 weeks to allow for tissue healing. Mobilization of the shoulder, using pendulum and circular exercises, is begun after that time. As shoulder motion improves, strengthening exercises for the rotator cuff muscles, the deltoid, and the biceps should be prescribed. If the athlete has 2 or more dislocations of the same shoulder joint, surgical repair should be considered.

Rotator Cuff Tear

Few tears of the rotator cuff are isolated lesions; they usually accompany a dislocation of the glenohumeral joint. They are usually caused by abducting the arm against resistance, such as in tackling or in wrestling. The prevalence of rotator cuff problems increases as age advances. There usually has been previous degeneration of the cuff when an active force completes the tear. Following the injury, there is difficulty in abducting the shoulder beyond 90 degrees without pain. The drop-arm test demonstrated in Figure 7–4 is positive. Chronic rotator cuff problems are discussed in more detail in Chapter 6.

The sore shoulder and arm are immobilized in a sling and ice packs applied. The rotator cuff tear normally heals with a conservative, nonoperative approach. Immobilization is necessary for 3 weeks, after which motion exercises are performed, followed by strengthening activities.

Acute Rupture of the Long Head of the Biceps

The biceps muscle has 2 tendons of origin (Fig 7–5). The short head originates from the coracoid process; the long head, originating from the rim of the glenoid, is inserted distally on the bicipital tuberosity of the radius. Rupture of the tendon occurs from forceful contraction of the muscles or from forced extension of the elbow with the biceps contracted. The musculotendinous unit may rupture either at its insertion point or

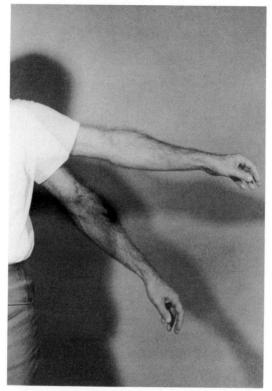

Fig 7–4.—Drop-arm test for torn rotator cuff. The patient's arm is elevated by the examiner and released. If the patient cannot sustain elevation, the rotator cuff is presumed to be torn.

in the belly of the muscle. The rupture occurs most commonly at the entrance of the long head of the biceps tendon into the bicipital groove of the humerus. The athlete complains of immediate pain and localized tenderness along the muscle. When the elbow is flexed, the biceps will roll up the front of the arm—the "popeye muscle."

Acute ruptures should be repaired surgically. Not repairing them causes some weakness of the arm, although elbow and shoulder motion usually will be normal.

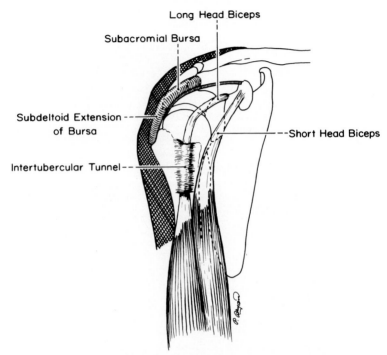

Fig 7–5. — Locations of the 2 tendons of the biceps shown in relation to the bursa of the shoulder.

Elbow

Dislocation of the Elbow

Dislocation of the elbow is caused by falling on the hyperextended elbow, and pushing the ulna out of its normal articulation with the distal humerus. The most common dislocation is posterolateral. Gross examination readily confirms the problem. The neurovascular structures distal to the elbow (Fig 7–6) must also be examined. Of particular importance is the quality of the radial pulse and the capillary filling of the fingernail beds. Particular attention must be paid to the median nerve, as well as the ulnar and radial nerve.

Reduction of the dislocation should be done as soon as possible, especially when there is nerve or vascular deficit. If the athlete is seen within minutes of the dislocation, it is often possible to reduce the elbow without any anesthesia by fixing the humerus with one hand and grasping the forearm, below the elbow, with the other, correcting the lateral displacement first. By applying gentle traction to the long axis of the joint, the coracoid process of the ulna can be brought gently anterior to the distal humerus, and the reduction accomplished. If it is impossible to reduce the elbow easily, the patient should be taken to a hospital where proper x-rays can be taken and adequate analgesia and muscle relaxation obtained. There is frequently a fracture of the humerus or the ulna associated with elbow dislocations. It is wise to get an x-ray, even if reduction has been accomplished without it, particularly in patients under 15, who still have open epiphysis around the elbow joint.

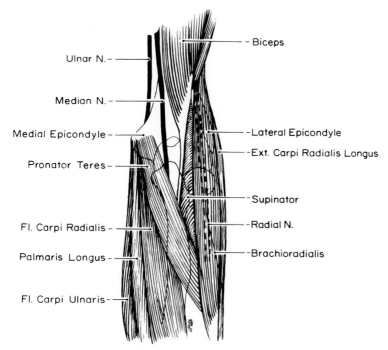

Fig 7–6.—Relationship of the nerves to the elbow joint demonstrates areas of potential nerve injury in elbow fractures and dislocations.

After reduction, the neurovascular structures should be reexamined. The elbow should be immobilized in a plaster cast or posterior plaster splint for 10 days with the forearm fully supinated and the elbow flexed to 90 degrees. For the next 10 days the posterior splint is removed intermittently and flexion exercises begun. After the splint is removed, active exercises are begun, but forceful, passive exercising is discouraged. Full motion may take many months to achieve, and elbow hyperextension may never be regained.

Fractures of the Elbow

Fractures of the elbow fortunately are not too common. Occasionally, they occur with dislocations. An elbow fracture can be very complicated to manage and should be referred to an orthopedist. The most frequent fracture around the elbow joint is a fracture of the radial head, occurring with a dislocated elbow or as an isolated problem. The athlete will have fallen on his outstretched arm, usually with more pressure on the radial side of the wrist, driving the radial head into the distal humerus and causing a fracture. Examination reveals tenderness over the radial head and probably limited supination and pronation. There is usually swelling within the radial humeral joint; however, diagnosis usually needs x-ray examination to be confirmed. A nondisplaced fracture of the radial head with full range of supination and pronation can be treated with sling immobilization for 10 days, followed by motion exercises. If there is any offset in the articulating surface of the radial head, or if more than 50% of the radial head is involved in the fracture, surgery may be necessary.

Injuries of the Forearm and Wrist

Fractures of the radius and ulna are probably the most common sports bone injuries, particularly in the younger athlete. A patient who has fallen on his outstretched hand and who complains about his wrist should be checked for fracture, particularly the younger athlete, where a greenstick or incomplete fracture can occur without creating any significant external deformity. A fracture of the radius and ulna, either in the shaft or in the distal area (Colles' fracture) usually is recognizable without x-rays. When such an injury is seen, the

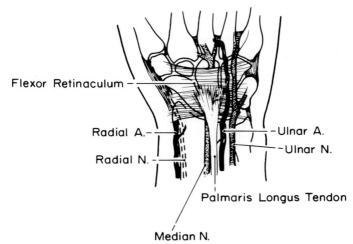

Flexor Retinaculum

Radial A.

Radial N.

Ulnar A.

Ulnar N.

Palmaris Longus Tendon

Median N.

Fig 7–7.—The palmaris longus provides the landmark for the median nerve at the wrist. The ulnar and radial arteries help locate the respective nerves. These relationships are important to evaluate possible injury, and these locations can also be utilized in regional anesthetic blocks.

circulation and the nerves should also be checked (Fig 7–7). X-ray views of the wrist and the elbow should be obtained. If only one bone is fractured, ligamentous injury involving either the proximal or distal radial-ulnar joint must be suspected.

The greenstick fracture can be safely treated with a cast or rigid splint, but any other fractures involving the radius and ulna should be referred to a specialist. Most fractures of the radius and ulna generally require a minimum of 6 weeks to heal.

Dislocations of the Wrist (Perilunate Transscaphoid)

Wrist dislocations occur from falling on the dorsiflexed wrist. The most common one is the lunate dislocation. Symptoms are pain in the wrist, dorsal swelling or fullness in the carpal tunnel area on palpation. X-rays are necessary to confirm the diagnosis; even with them the perilunate dislocation, which is often subtle, is frequently missed. In the lunate dislocation the lunate has been squeezed and rotated into the volar area of the wrist. In the perilunar dislocation, the lunate maintains its normal anatomic relationship with the radius and the remainder of the carpal bones are dislocated. Many times "things just don't look right" on the x-rays, but the exact anatomical delineation may escape the inexperienced observer.

The dislocation, lunar or perilunar, must be reduced as soon as possible. With the perilunar dislocation there may be an associated fracture of the navicular, and 5–6 weeks of immobilization for a dislocation is extended to a number of months (see below).

Fracture of the Navicular

Navicular fractures are probably the most missed diagnosis concerning the musculoskeletal system. The athlete will have fallen on his wrist. There is pain, frequently localized to the radial side of the wrist, but often generalized and limited motion. The principal symptom, however, is tenderness in the anatomical "snuff box," that area located on the thumb side of the wrist between the extensor and abductor tendons to the thumb. Tenderness in that area, even with normal x-rays, may indicate a fractured navicular.

Because this is a commonly missed diagnosis and because delay in treatment often compromises results, treatment must proceed without a confirmed diagnosis. When there is tenderness in the "snuff box," even though x-rays are normal, the injured wrist and hand should be immobilized in a thumb spica for 10 days to 2 weeks. When the cast is removed, more x-rays should be taken. If there is a navicular fracture, the body mechanisms will have cleaned up the debris along the fracture line, making it radiolucent on x-ray; this establishes the diagnosis. The thumb spica must be kept in place until healing is complete, which may take 6 months to a year. Treatment of the ununited navicular fracture is discussed in Chapter 6.

Wrist Sprains

Next to ankle sprains, wrist sprains are the most common musculoskeletal injury in athletes. They are usually caused by falling on the outstretched hand. In a first-degree sprain there is soreness but very little swelling. In a second-degree sprain there is swelling, and discomfort on range of motion. In the third-degree sprain the wrist is unstable. X-rays should be obtained to rule out a carpal bone dislocation or a fracture of the navicular.

First-degree sprains often need only limited rest with elevation to control swelling. Second-degree sprains need external support from a wrist splint for at least 10 days, after which early motion can begin. Full external support should be maintained for 3 weeks, after which time range of motion and strengthening of the forearm musculature can be advised. Third-degree sprains need to be immobilized for approximately 4 weeks, followed by another 2 weeks of external support with some active mobility exercises being done intermittently. Subsequently, forearm muscle strengthening exercises can be started. There are very few indications for surgery in wrist ligament problems without an associated carpal bone injury or fracture. Third-degree injuries may require a specialist's consultation.

Hands and Fingers

Fractures of the Metacarpals and Phalanges

Fractures of the metacarpals and phalanges occur in many ways. The hand may be stepped on, it may be caught between two objects or it may strike an object. All produce fractures of varying degrees of displacement, angulation and severity that are indicated by some anatomical disalignment, pain at the fracture site, crepitus and loss of function. When anatomical alignment is normal, compression in the long axis of the bone will often cause pain at the fracture site. X-rays of all injuries should be obtained.

Fractures of the fingers can run the gamut from very easy to most difficult to treat. Discussion here will be limited to those that are easy to treat. All others should be referred to an orthopedist. A transverse or slightly oblique fracture of the metacarpal shaft without displacement can be treated with a short arm cast for 3 weeks. If the metacarpal fracture is at the head of the fourth or fifth finger (boxer's fracture), treatment is more difficult. If there is more than 30 degrees angular deformity at the fracture site, reduction must be done. Angulation of less than 30 degrees can be treated with further protection if the athlete realizes he will "lose" that knuckle, although there should be no functional loss. Reduction of the sharply angulated boxer's fracture requires a local anesthetic and a special casting position, which needs to be maintained for about 10 days. Longer maintenance in this hypercorrected position produces joint stiffness that is difficult to overcome. This fracture should probably be managed by an orthopedic surgeon.

Treatment of fractures involving the shaft of the phalanges, if they are transverse and aligned anatomically, can be done by splinting the finger with 10–15 degrees of flexion at each joint for approximately 2 weeks. If the finger feels stable, dynamic splinting can be started by taping the injured finger to the adjacent one. It should be maintained with this dynamic splinting for another 10 days. Splinting may then be discontinued, except for taping the 2 fingers together for any type of physical activity for an additional 3–4 weeks. If the fracture is oblique with any shortening, extends into the joint or is otherwise unstable, it should be referred to an orthopedist. In fractures of the distal phalanx, usually crushing, management of the soft tissue injury is all that is required.

Dislocations of the Fingers

There are 4 principal dislocations of the fingers. The 2 most common ones are dislocation of the metacarpal phalangeal joint of the thumb and dislocation of the proximal interphalangeal joints of any of the fingers. Two less frequent dislocations are those of the metacarpal phalangeal joints of the index finger, and of the distal interphalangeal joints of the fingers. The athlete with interphalangeal joint dislocations, whether proximal or distal, may take it upon himself to reduce the dislocation. Often the trainer performs that service. X-rays should still be obtained to rule out any unrecognized fracture or interarticular problem. Regardless of who did the reduction, the injury should be treated by a physician (see below).

If traction at the time of injury has not reduced the dislocation, some type of local anesthetic will be required to relax the muscle sufficiently. Traction on the joint in the long axis, while applying gentle pressure over the dislocated bone, will

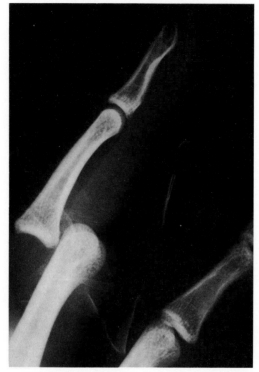

Fig 7–8. — Dislocation of the proximal interphalangeal joint.

affect the reduction. Dislocation at the metacarpal phalangeal joint, particularly the index finger, may be unreducible by normal methods. In this instance the metacarpal head dislocates through the ligamentous structures, becomes locked and an open reduction is necessary. Occasionally at the proximal interphalangeal joint the volar plate will become impinged dorsally, acting as a block to reduction by the normal methods. Open reduction will be necessary.

Following reduction, 10 days of immobilization, using a splint, are necessary (Fig 7–8 and 7–9). When the splint is removed, the injured joint, particularly the proximal interphalangeal joint, should be reexamined. Two significant problems can arise: boutonnière deformity (discussed below) and

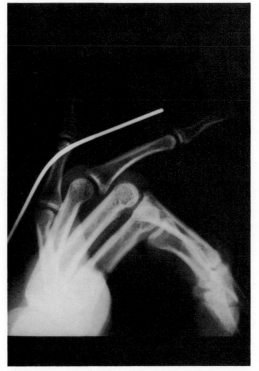

Fig 7–9.—Postreduction of a dislocated proximal interphalangeal joint with splint immobilization.

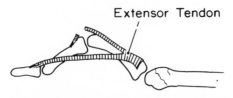

Extensor Tendon

Fig 7–10.—Boutonnière deformity. Rupture at the insertion of the extensor tendon's central slip allows herniation of the proximal interphalangeal joint dorsally between the lateral slips.

an injury to the volar plate, through the fibrous portion. If the volar plate is examined with a blunt instrument, localized tenderness in the proximal portion indicates that continued volar plate healing is necessary. Static splinting should be resumed. If there is no evidence of the boutonnière deformity or of volar plate injury, dynamic splinting (taping to the adjacent finger) should be maintained for 10 days and then discontinued. For any type of athletic activity involving contact, splinting to the adjacent finger should continue for another 3 weeks. When applying a static splint to any finger injury, it is best to immobilize only the injured joint, leaving the other joints free to maintain the range of motion.

Rupture of the Extensor Central Slip (Boutonnière Deformity)

Dislocations of the proximal interphalangeal joint often create injuries to the central slip of the extensor tendon. The common extensor to each finger courses as one tendon over the metacarpal phalangeal joint. As it approaches the proximal interphalangeal joint, it splits into 3 slips. One inserts at the base of the middle phalanx over the joint; one courses radially, the other ulnarly; the 2 then course dorsally to unite in the midline over the middle phalanx. Rupture of the attachment of the central slip on the dorsal side of the middle phalanx creates a "buttonhole" or boutonnière deformity (Fig 7–10). Because of swelling and generalized soreness, this injury is often missed. Localized tenderness at the point of insertion indicates a potential boutonnière problem.

This injury should be treated on suspicion. X-rays are usually normal. Since the deformity is caused by rupture of the central slip, treatment methods relax the tendon so that the central slip can be approximated to its point of insertion. If the splint is applied so that the proximal interphalangeal joint is held in full extension to hyperextension, the distal phalangeal joint should be allowed free movement. This position relaxes the central slip of the extensor tendon. This method of treatment, even in experienced hands, is often unsuccessful, and this injury probably should be referred to an orthopedic or a hand surgeon. If the injury is diagnosed early, surgical repair gives the best results.

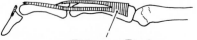

Extensor   Tendon
Fig 7–11. — Rupture of extensor tendon distally.

Rupture of the Extensor Tendon Distally (Mallet Finger, Baseball Finger)

Striking the tip of a finger with an object such as a baseball can produce 3 injuries. Dislocation of a phalangeal joint was discussed previously. Either occurring with this dislocation or as an isolated problem is fracture of the distal phalanx on the dorsal side. This disrupts the common extensor tendon to the distal phalanx (Fig 7–11). The extensor tendon may also be torn without any associated fracture, producing the same problem, i.e., a dropped distal phalanx. The athlete complains of soreness over the distal interphalangeal joint dorsally, is unable to extend that joint actively and has a flexion deformity of 15–45 degrees. X-rays should be taken to confirm the presence of a fracture. If a fracture involves more than one third of the articular surface of the distal phalanx, surgery will be necessary. A fracture involving less than one third can be treated nonoperatively by the experienced surgeon.

The distal interphalangeal joint must be splinted in an extension or slight hyperextension for 6–8 weeks. An internal splint, using a pin, can be used to maintain the distal phalangeal joint in full extension. Splinting at night should continue for 3–6 additional weeks. Management of this problem can be difficult in inexperienced hands, and referral is often the wisest course.

Rupture of the Flexor Tendon

Tackling in football or weightlifting can cause a rupture of a flexor tendon to a digit. The most frequently ruptured tendon is the flexor digitorum profundus, usually to the long finger, but occasionally to the index or ring digit. The athlete frequently does not remember when the injury occurred, but notices the finger does not quite "work right." It may take careful examination to reveal abnormal function of the profundus. To test this the proximal interphalangeal joint of the injured finger is maintained in full extension by the examiner. The athlete should be able to flex the distal phalanx 45–60 degrees with good strength. With a rupture of the profundus the strength is lost, if not the motion. To confirm the diagnosis, range and strength can be compared with the opposite finger.

Splinting, which can be done successfully in extensor tendon injuries, will not work here. An open repair is necessary, and referral to a hand surgeon is recommended.

Nail Injuries

The fingernail has two parts. The sterile matrix is the distal portion and is pink in color. It functions as a smooth surface on which the nail grows. The more proximal portion of the nail bed is the germinal matrix, which causes the nail to grow. The skin overlying the base of the nail is called the eponychium, and the skin on either border is the paronychium (Fig 7–12).

Subungual Hematoma

The most common injury to the nail is the subungual hematoma. If the nail bed is discolored but the injury is not painful, nothing needs to be done. Frequently, the athlete complains of a throbbing pain, almost as if he can feel his heart beat. Oc-

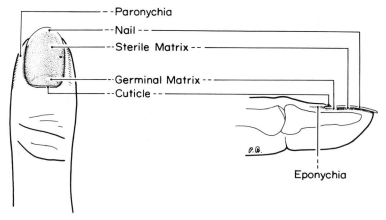

Fig 7–12.—Structure of the nail bed.

casionally, x-rays are indicated to check for a distal tuft fracture.

Elevating the hand and placing ice on the finger may help.
Often, it is necessary to relieve the hematoma with a small
hole in the nail bed. This can be made by heating a paper clip
over an alcohol lamp and gently burning a hole through the
nail. It is not necessary to remove the nail.

Nail Avulsion

Nail avulsions occur most frequently in contact sports. The
nail may be partially or completely avulsed from the base on
either the radial or the ulnar side. If the avulsion has caused a
laceration of the nail bed, the eponychium or paronychium, it
should be repaired surgically. If the base of the nail has been
avulsed from the bed of the germinal matrix, only the base
should be excised, leaving the remainder intact. In general, it
is best to leave any part of the nail that is still smooth and attached. The laceration of the nail bed should be minimally
debrided and repaired with very fine catgut. In a laceration
extending into the eponychium, the free edges of the eponychium must be approximated or the edges will scar to the germinal matrix, preventing normal nail growth.

Human Bite

Although it is not truly a human bite, a laceration produced
when the fist strikes the human tooth should be treated as
such. Without proper treatment, an infection that is difficult to
treat may result.

Under good lighting the wound should be washed and all
contused and necrotic tissue excised. The extensor tendon
mechanism should be inspected with the finger in both full
flexion and full extension. Any tendon laceration should be
repaired. Skin edges should be thoroughly debrided and then
carefully approximated. It may be wise to put a small wick in
the wound to allow for drainage. If the wick is not used, the
patient should be seen within 24 hours and again within 48
hours to check for developing infections. Apply an aluminum
or plaster splint to the damaged finger. If there are no tendon
injuries, the sutures can be removed in about 10 days and
splinting discontinued. If the tendon has been injured, the
finger should be splinted for an additional week.

Pelvis, Hip and Thigh

Contusion

A contusion of the thigh is a frequent injury in contact sports, particularly football. Usually the athlete can remember being hit but is not disabled at the time. He will continue to play and then complain of soreness, usually in the anterior thigh. Examination reveals diffuse tenderness, usually in the midportion of the quadriceps. Flexion of the knee beyond 90 degrees will put the anterior thigh muscles under tension and cause discomfort.

Swelling may indicate a hematoma deep within the thigh. Under the very strictest aseptic conditions an aspiration can be attempted. The limb should be elevated. Ice and compression should be applied. If the swelling is marked and the pain is severe, the patient should be given a pair of crutches and advised not to bear weight on the injured limb. He should be checked within 24–48 hours and the ice, elevation and immobilization continued. At 48–72 hours, heat, in the form of a whirlpool bath, can be substituted for ice. Activity can be resumed as discomfort allows. Athletes should not be returned to competition until all swelling has resolved and there is no tenderness on light activity. Returning to activity too soon or sustaining a reinjury may cause myositis ossificans.

Hip Pointer

Avulsion of a part of the muscle attached to the iliac crest produces a hip pointer. This is usually caused by a direct blow to the area. The athlete is unable to move without discomfort in the area, which becomes worse with running. Examination shows tenderness localized along the crest of the ilium. The pathology is a tear of a portion of the lower abdominal or pelvic muscles from the ilium. Seldom does avulsion of a portion of the iliac crest occur.

This injury should be treated like other strains. The area should be rested by putting the athlete on crutches. Ice should be applied during the first 24–48 hours and heat introduced at about 72 hours. The athlete should be kept on crutches until he is reasonably comfortable walking. Activities should be gauged by the amount of discomfort. Contact sports should not be resumed until all soreness is gone. It is probably wise to pad the injured area for several weeks after resumption of activities. It is not unusual for this injury to take 4–6 weeks to resolve.

Dislocated Hip

Dislocation of the hip, an unusual injury in athletics, is more likely to occur in the younger athlete. The diagnosis is usually obvious. Posterior dislocation is the most common occurrence. The leg will be seen in an attitude of internal rotation and adduction with some flexion. Any motion will be very painful.

The athlete should be carefully transported from the playing area and taken to the nearest hospital. X-rays and a neurological examination should be done prior to reduction. A general anesthetic will be required for reduction, which should be done as soon as possible.

Fractured Femur

A fractured femur is also not common in sports because the femur requires a great amount of force in order to be fractured. When it does occur, the athlete is immediately disabled and the diagnosis is usually obvious. The leg should be splinted, preferably with some type of caliper device, but a piece of material that reaches from the greater trochanter to the toes will suffice.

The patient should be admitted to the hospital under the care of a specialist. Since this injury is more common in the younger athlete, definitive treatment will probably consist of traction for 6 weeks followed by a body spica cast for another 6 weeks. In adults the fracture can be treated with open reduction and internal fixation.

Knee

Fractures about the Knee

There are four significant fractures involving the knee that should be mentioned. They are fracture of the patella, fracture of the tibial plateau, avulsion of the tibial spine and fracture of the tibial tubercle. Fractures about the patella occur either through the upper pole, through the lower pole or through the medial and lateral edges. The athlete complains of soreness and some swelling about the knee. Usually there is dysfunction of the extensor mechanism. In a complete separation of the extensor mechanism, a defect can be felt within the body of the patella. X-rays will be needed to confirm the fracture and to aid proper treatment. It is important for the inexperienced to recognize the entity called a bipartite patella, which is an anatomical variant where the patella is composed of 2 parts. It should not be mistaken for an acute fracture.

The other fracture involving the extensor mechanism is avulsion of the tibial tubercle. The patellar tendon attaches to the tibia on the tubercle. If an athlete gets his leg in a position that concentrates all the weight on the attachment of the tibial tendon at the tibial tubercle, there may be localized tenderness and swelling, together with weakness of the extensor mechanism due to pain and loss of integrity. X-rays are needed to distinguish the patellar tendon rupture from tibial tubercle avulsion.

Fracture of the tibial plateau, either medial or lateral, occurs when the athlete is caught off balance and compressive forces are exerted on either the medial or lateral compartment, creating compression of the plateau. The athlete complains of tenderness and swelling in the knee on weight bearing and a feeling of instability. X-rays are needed to delineate the extent of tibial plateau compression.

The fourth fracture is avulsion of the tibial spine. In reality, this is similar to a tear of the anterior cruciate, as that ligament attaches to the tibia on the tibial spine. There will be swelling within the knee joint, tenderness and probably some anterior instability, which is often difficult to identify because the intra-articular fracture produces a hemarthrosis. The marked swelling tends to obviate the instability. X-rays show a pull-off fracture of the tibial spine.

Treatment of all these fractures is best handled by an orthopedic surgeon. Of the four, the avulsion of the tibial spine with the attached cruciate ligament is the only one that is frequently treated by closed methods. The intra-articular hematoma can be aspirated, the joint anesthetized with an analgesic and the knee placed in full extension, often reducing the avul-

sion. Immobilizing the knee in a cylinder cast in slight hyperextension can be effective treatment; however, this decision
should be made by an orthopedic surgeon.

Dislocations about the Knee

There are two dislocations of significance around the knee
joint. One is a dislocation of the entire knee joint, and the
other is a dislocation of the patella. Dislocation of the knee
joint requires a great amount of force and is thus considered
rare in athletics. However, it is more common than thought,
but it goes unrecognized. In most instances where there has
been a tear of the cruciates associated with tear of the collateral
ligament, there is at least some subluxation. Thus if one includes subluxation, this problem is more common than recognized. Dislocations can occur in any direction, but the most
frequent is an anterior dislocation produced by forced hyperextension of the knee. After recognizing that the knee has
been dislocated, the physician must determine the vascular
integrity distal to the knee. In either the anterior or the posterior dislocation, a significant tear of an artery can occur. Failure to recognize this may jeopardize the viability of the leg.
Checking the dorsalis pedis pulse and the posterior tibial
pulse are of prime importance. An arteriogram may be necessary to delineate the vascular supply.

Dislocation of the patella is caused by excessive lateral
force on the patellar extensor mechanism, which tears the
medial muscular and capsular structures. The patella dislocates laterally. If the athlete is seen at the time of injury the
patella will frequently be in its dislocated position. If any time
has lapsed, the patella may be relocated. The first person to
see the athlete usually tries to extend the knee, and if pain and
muscle spasm has not already interceded the patella may slide
back medially. If the patella is in its usual position at the time
of the examination, the athlete will have tenderness along its
medial border and swelling in that area. He will be very reluc-
tant to allow the examiner to attempt to move the patella laterally. These factors are almost pathognomonic of a reduced dislocated patella. X-rays should be taken to confirm the dislocation if the patella is still out of place. If it is not, associated in-

juries or an avulsion of the patella's medial edge need to be determined.

Treatment of both these dislocations is often surgical, although there is some difference of opinion among orthopedists about treatment methods. Many think that a dislocation can be reduced and treated in a cylinder cast in extension. However, for a fracture through the medial edge of the patella, most agree that the treatment of choice is surgery.

Muscle Tendon Ruptures

We have already stated that the extensor mechanism of the knee can be disrupted at its insertion on the tibial tubercle or disrupted by fractures through the patella. A third extensor mechanism disruption occurs with rupture of the quadriceps tendon or muscle, usually at the insertion on the superior pole of the patella. It may be associated with a pull-off fracture of the superior pole. All extensor tendon injuries are caused by an unexpected flexion force resisted by a sudden reflex contraction of the quadriceps. The rupture can be complete or incomplete. With a complete rupture the patient cannot actively extend the knee. Passive extension is possible, but painful. A defect can often be palpated above the patella. With an incomplete rupture, swelling and generalized tenderness may cause tears to go undiagnosed. Careful palpation, with the quadriceps actively contracted, may reveal such an injury.

The incomplete rupture may be treated conservatively by splinting in extension for 14–21 days and then gradually mobilizing the knee. Treatment of the complete rupture is surgical.

Tears of the Meniscus or Semilunar Cartilages

Semilunar cartilages are frequently injured in contact sports. The medial meniscus (Fig 7–13) is more frequently injured for 2 reasons. First, the medial meniscus has less mobility because of firmer attachment along its borders. Second, there is a greater opportunity for forces to be applied from the side to the flexed, loaded knee with the foot firmly planted. This force on the medial meniscus produces 1 of 3 types of tears: (1), a bucket-handle tear in which the central portion of the cartilage is torn and dislocated into the intercondylar

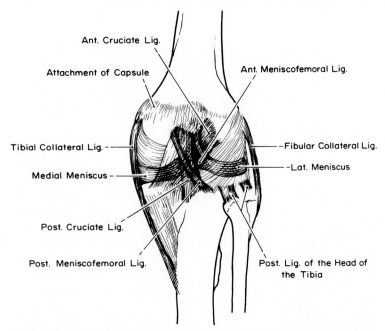

Ant. Cruciate Lig.

Attachment of Capsule

Ant. Meniscofemoral Lig.

Tibial Collateral Lig.

Fibular Collateral Lig.

Medial Meniscus

Lat. Meniscus

Post. Cruciate Lig.

Post. Meniscofemoral Lig.

Post. Lig. of the Head of the Tibia

Fig 7–13.—Knee anatomy, posterior view. The relationship of the cartilages and various ligaments helps the physician to understand the physical findings in knee injuries.

notch, creating a locked knee or a knee that will not flex or extend; (2), a tear of the anterior attachment of the meniscus, which allows the anterior horn to float into the internal part of the knee, preventing full extension; and (3) a detachment of the posterior horn, which will often produce a feeling of instability when the athlete puts weight on the slightly flexed knee.

Examination reveals swelling and generalized tenderness along the joint line, most frequently the medial line. The knee may not flex or extend more than a few degrees, or there may be a block to full extension with normal flexion. McMurray's test will often be positive. This test is performed by putting the knee in a flexed position, then gradually extending and externally rotating the tibia on the femur. A positive result, a palpable or audible click in the medial joint space (often painful), is fairly strong evidence of torn cartilage. X-rays, however, are usually normal. The recently developed arthrogram technique, in which a small amount of dye and air is instilled into the knee joint, frequently shows the location of the tear. Although the diagnosis may not be obvious, there occasionally is a tear of the other meniscus, which can be shown by an arthrogram. This is important to know preoperatively.

Once a diagnosis of torn cartilage has been made, surgical removal is indicated. Another diagnostic test that can be done just before arthrotomy is an arthroscopic exam. It can be done instead of, or in addition to, the arthrogram to delineate an injury other than the suspected torn cartilage. Following removal of the meniscus, the orthopedic surgeon will instruct the athlete in regaining full range of motion, particularly extension and strengthening the quadriceps. In the uncomplicated cartilage removal, this will require about 6 weeks.

Tears of the Cruciate Ligaments

An isolated tear of the anterior cruciate can occur when force is directed toward the tibia from behind. The posterior cruciate is torn by force directed to the proximal portion of the tibia in the posterior direction (see Fig 7–13). In athletes, the anterior cruciate tear is more common. The patient with such a tear may complain of feelings of instability (e.g., that the knee will "give way"), particularly on going up or down stairs. Examination shows a painful, swollen knee with limited motion. The drawer sign, described previously in Chapter 6, should be tested. A positive result indicates a tear of the cruciate that should be treated immediately; late reconstruction is difficult.

This injury should be treated by an orthopedic surgeon. Some orthopedists think that the ligaments should be surgically repaired; others recommend application of a cylinder cast for 6 weeks followed by intensive quadriceps strengthening exercises.

Collateral Ligament Sprains

Medial collateral ligament injuries are far more common than lateral collateral ligament injuries (see Fig 7–13). In sports such as football and skiing, there is ample opportunity for the knee to be extended and have an abduction force applied to the tibial collateral ligament, causing a stretching or tearing of the ligament. A first-degree sprain causes some soreness and minimal swelling along the injured ligament. With a second-degree injury there may also be ecchymosis and more intense tenderness. In the third-degree injury the knee is unstable. It may be difficult to distinguish a tear of the ligament from a tear of the meniscus. In more severe injuries, it may be necessary to examine the knee under anesthesia in order to arrive at the correct diagnosis. In conjunction with an examination under anesthesia, it may be beneficial to obtain stress x-ray views of the knee.

Normally, first- and second-degree strains can be treated by ice, elevation and immobilization. Second-degree injuries require a longer period of immobilization—usually at least 6 weeks. Third-degree injuries require surgical repair. In many instances it is wisest and safest to refer second-degree injuries also.

The Unhappy Triad

The unhappy triad, named by Dr. Donald O'Donoghue, combines 3 injuries—tears of the anterior cruciate, the medial collateral ligament and the medial meniscus. Massive knee injuries require a high level of expertise, not only in diagnosis but in treatment.

Early diagnosis and repair gives the best results. Treatment by a specialist is imperative.

Leg and Ankle

Fractures

Fracture of the long bones of the leg is an occasional occurrence in athletics. Examination of the athlete with a fractured tibia or fibula reveals an abnormal anatomical alignment, swelling, tenderness and crepitus at the fracture site. More frequently, the ankle is fractured and dislocated simultaneously. Symptoms are abnormal anatomical alignment, swelling, tenderness, occasional discoloration, pain and instability. X-ray examination is necessary.

All fractures, no matter how severe, require casting; most require reduction.

Sprain of the Ankle

Ankle sprain (Fig 7–14) is by far the most common sports injury to the lower extremity. In a second-degree injury, in addition to tenderness and swelling, there is some restriction of motion. What motion there is usually is painful. X-rays should be taken to rule out associated bone injuries. The third-degree sprain, in addition to the above physical findings, is also characterized by some instability of the ankle mortice. If there is any question, stress views of the ankle joint should be ordered to confirm the instability.

Treatment of the first-degree sprain is symptomatic. Elevation and ice are recommended. Activity should be determined by the comfort level. Once the symptoms subside, the athlete may return to normal activity. For a second-degree sprain, support from a splint or cast will be necessary for 14–21 days. Examination should be repeated to determine residual prob-

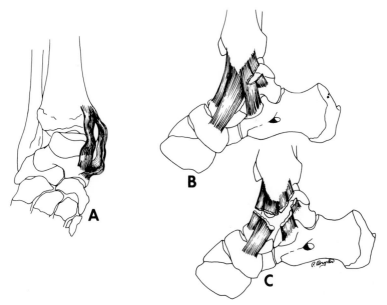

Fig 7–14. — Ankle sprains. **A,** first-degree sprain of the deltoid ligament. **B,** second-degree sprain of the tibial talar ligament. **C,** third-degree sprain of the medial ligaments.

lems. If there is still significant swelling and discomfort with manipulation of the joint, an additional 2–3 weeks of immobilization will produce better healing. When the cast is removed, gradual mobilization of the joint is begun, followed by strengthening exercises for the dorsiflexors, plantar flexors, invertors and evertors of the foot and ankle. A third-degree sprain may require surgical repair of the torn ligaments. This decision should be made by an orthopedic surgeon.

Anterior Tibial Compartment Syndrome

Any entity that causes swelling in the anterior compartment of the leg can produce a syndrome. The initial complaint is usually severe pain, followed by loss of function of the anterior tibial muscle, the extensor hallucis muscle and the extensor digitorum longus muscles, all in the anterior compartment. This functional loss results in a dropped foot. The most frequent cause of this problem is a direct blow over the anterior compartment; other causes may be infection or strenuous use. In extreme cases the peroneal nerve may be compromised, causing loss of sensation over the lateral leg. X-rays usually are not helpful.

Because the results of treatment delay are so drastic, the anterior compartment should be decompressed surgically upon suspicion.

Peroneal Nerve Contusion

The peroneal nerve, as it winds behind the head of the fibula just below the knee joint, is frequently exposed to injury, usually from a direct blow over the head of the fibula. The first symptom is usually a lightening-like pain, followed by tingling or paresthesia along the side of the leg. Examination may reveal swelling around the head of the fibula. Tapping over this area will produce paresthesia in the distribution of the peroneal nerve.

If there is no associated laceration, the physician can be fairly certain that the nerve is in continuity. Therefore, observation is usually all that is necessary. If the patient develops a foot drop, support of the extremity in a short leg cast or a brace may be necessary until the nerve begins to recover. Usually it will do so. Progress of recovery can be followed by tapping over the course of the nerve to locate the regenerating neuroma (Tinel's test).

Rupture of the Achilles Tendon

The Achilles tendon rupture is an injury frequently seen in athletes who participate in sports played with a racquet. The athlete will describe planting his foot, putting all his weight on the foot and feeling something "give" in his ankle. This is followed by immediate pain in the posterior lower leg. The athlete is unable to run because he cannot push off. Examination shows tenderness and swelling, usually not at the insertion of the Achilles tendon on the os calcis, but an inch or so proximal. Sometimes there will be a palpable defect. The squeeze test, performed by vigorously squeezing the calf muscle, will be positive. Normally, this produces plantar flexion of the foot, but not in rupture of the Achilles tendon. X-rays should be taken, as the tendon will occasionally pull off with a small fragment of the os calcis. This factor influences the method of treatment.

The preferred method of treatment is probably open repair of the tendon. However, for the mature athlete who is competing for fun alone, an open repair may not be indicated. Good results have been obtained by applying a plaster cast with the knee flexed approximately 30 degrees and with the foot and ankle plantar flexed 35–40 degrees. This position is maintained for about 3 weeks, when the knee portion of the cast is removed. The healing Achilles tendon is protected for about 8 weeks in a cast. Once the cast is removed the patient is allowed to walk with an elevated heel, gradually decreasing the elevation over several months. When the Achilles tendon is fully stretched, normal activities can be resumed.

Rupture of the Plantaris

The plantaris is a small muscle that lies parallel to the gastro-soleus muscle and tendon. It is frequently ruptured in the athlete aged 35 or older who participates in racket sports. The athlete has acute pain in the calf, followed by soreness. Often the athlete continues to play but eventually the soreness makes play impossible. There is no functional loss. Examination is often unrevealing. There may be localized tenderness at the junction of the proximal and middle third of the leg posteriorly.

Treatment is symptomatic only. The heel can be elevated half an inch to an inch to make walking more comfortable. Ice can be applied to acute injuries, followed by heat 48–72 hours later. Activity is dictated by comfort. Symptoms generally subside in 6 weeks.

The Foot

Fractures

Fractures are usually caused by direct trauma, such as getting stepped on. Exam reveals swelling and tenderness over the fracture site. X-rays should be obtained. Immobilization in a cast for about 3 weeks is usually necessary. If the phalanges are anatomically aligned to the naked eye, strapping to the adjacent toe may be all that is required. Occasionally fractures of the great toe require a cast to maintain alignment.

Dislocations of the Toes

Dislocations of the toes are not too common; they occur most frequently at the distal interphalangeal joint. There is usually anatomical disalignment, and x-rays confirm the dislocation.

Reduction can often be accomplished without anesthesia. If not, an analgesic should be injected in the web on either side of the injured toe. Very rarely will it be necessary to reduce the joint surgically.

SUGGESTED READING

1. Adams, J. C.: *Outline of Orthopedics* (Baltimore: Williams & Wilkins Co., 1971).
2. Care, E. F., Burke, J. F., and Boyd, R. S.: *Trauma Management* (Chicago: Year Book Medical Publishers, Inc., 1974).
3. Hoppenfeld, S.: *Physical Examination of the Spine and Extremities* (New York: Appleton Century Crofts, 1976).
4. *Introduction to Sports Medicine* (Cleveland: Case Western Reserve University Press, 1976).
5. O'Donoghue, D. H.: *Treatment of Injuries to Athletes* (Philadelphia: W. B. Saunders Co., 1976).

6. Rockwood, C. J. and Green, D. P.: *Fractures,* Vol. 1 and 2 (Philadelphia: J. B. Lippincott, 1975).

7. *Orthopedic Clinics of North America,* Vol. 4, (Philadelphia: W. B. Saunders Co., 1973).

8. Watson-Jones: *Fractures and Joint Injuries,* Vol. 1 and 2 (Edinburgh: Churchill Livingston, 1965).

8 / Evaluation of the Young Athlete

During the past two decades, children's sports programs have grown tremendously. Little leagues have been formed in almost every conceivable sport. With this much activity, a participating youngster is going to sustain injuries. In evaluating these injuries the physician must remember that the junior-league body is growing, developing and, to some extent, uncoordinated. Problems different from those seen in adults will be encountered.

The young musculoskeletal system has different proportions from the adult's. The head is larger in comparison to the rest of the skeleton. More rapid growth of the appendicular and axial skeleton occurs later, leaving the skull smaller. During the first 6–12 years, the child will average about 2½ inches per year of growth, mostly in the long bones, and will gain approximately 7 pounds per year.

Nutrition requirements are different. For instance, children aged 7–9 require approximately 80 calories per kilogram of body weight, around 3 grams of protein per kilogram and 75 milliliters of water per kilogram. Comparable adult values are 40 calories per kilogram, 1 gram of protein per kilogram and 50 milliliters of water per kilogram daily. In order for the child to achieve his growth potential, he must receive sufficient food and fluid both to grow and to maintain athletic activity.

A WORD OF ADVICE

There will often be undue pressure on both the physician and the young athlete to return an injured player sooner than may be judicious. An overzealous parent or coach, or occasionally an athlete, may not permit the injury to run its course. Because of the publicity given athletic injuries, parents and coaches know that professional athletes can recuperate from different injuries in a specific length of time. They often expect youngsters to do the same. No athletic season, and certainly no athletic contest, is important enough to jeopardize the career of a potentially good athlete by expecting performance before the body has recovered from an injury. In the realm of children's sports there is certainly no place for "playing hurt."

FRACTURES

Fractures are more common in the youth or adolescent than in adults. The activities of youth are more carefree. Children's bones are more slender. The fracture in the youth, however, has one treatment advantage that the adult fracture does not: the bone will undergo remodeling. A growing bone is divided into several parts (Fig 8 – 1). As long as the epiphyseal plate is open, there is some growth potential. When a bone with growth potential is broken, a fracture may heal with anatomical disalignment. As growth progresses, there is deposition of bone along the lines of stress with resorption of bone where no stress is applied. This allows for complete anatomical realignment following healing.

Fractures in children heal more rapidly. For instance, the femoral shaft fracture occurring at age 8, will be united in about 2 months. At age 12, it will take approximately 10 weeks and after the age of 20 it will take 3 – 4 months.

Another special problem peculiar to children's fractures is length or growth aberration. If the epiphyseal plate is injured, either totally or partially, the growth potential of the bone can be altered. This creates either a progressive angulation deformity or shortness of the extremity. Thus, whenever a fracture involves the growth area, the athlete and his family must be forewarned of the potential for growth disturbances as the youngster matures.

After x-ray evaluation to determine the exact extent of damage, as accurate a reduction as possible should be done. This

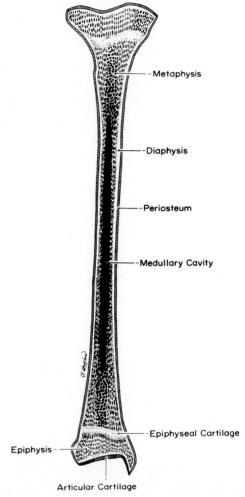

Fig 8–1.—A typical bone in a growing child. As long as the epiphyseal cartilage line is present, the bone has growth potential and can remodel after fracture.

is followed by immobilization in a plaster cast for the appropriate length of time. There are very few indications for open reduction of fractures in the youth or adolescent. Specific indications for surgery are femoral neck fractures, some epiphyseal injuries and certain displaced interarticular fractures. Even though it sounds as if treatment of youth and adolescent fractures may be less demanding than adult fractures, the only fracture that should be treated by the inexperienced physician is the incomplete, or greenstick, fracture. This injury requires protective immobilization, usually for 3 weeks, perhaps longer in some lower-extremity fractures.

UPPER EXTREMITY PROBLEMS

Clavicle Fractures

The clavicle is probably the most frequently broken bone in the youth. It heals readily and rapidly. Treatment consists of immobilization in a figure-8 bandage and hyperabducting the shoulders. A sling for the arm on the side of the injured clavicle enhances comfort. Parents should be warned that prominence at the healing fracture site may be evident, but usually remodeling will reduce the size of the prominence over time.

Elbow Fractures

The most serious and complicated fracture and/or dislocation in the upper extremity involves the elbow. There are multiple growth centers around the elbow which, if injured, can create growth problems. Fortunately this does not occur frequently. Treatment of elbow injuries should be managed by a specialist.

Little Leaguer's Elbow

Complaints of pain along the medial aspect of the elbow related to throwing have been described as "little leaguer's elbow." This is produced by throwing excessively, by throwing a curve ball or by using a maneuver that produces a snapping of the wrist or elbow during execution. A traction problem is created on the attachments of the flexor muscle mass over the medial epicondyle at the elbow. Repetition of such motions applies stress to the attachments of these muscles at the growth line of the apophysis. Inflammation results; pain and localized swelling ensue. Examination shows localized tenderness and soft tissue swelling in the region of the medial epicondyle. X-rays may show some widening of the epiphyseal plate and soft tissue swelling.

Treatment consists of curtailing whatever activities have produced the soreness until the pain has disappeared. This may involve restriction of activities for an entire season or year. When the symptoms have cleared, forearm-strengthening exercises, using light weights, will help rebuild the forearm and may prevent recurrence.

In the early days of little league baseball, this problem was so common that a rule was introduced that disallowed pitching and catching for more than 3 consecutive innings. The amount of practice throwing also was restricted. It is now recognized that the amount of throwing that will produce an elbow problem in one child may not produce it in another. Many people think that penalizing all youth because of the problem some may develop is not right. However, there is no adequate way to determine in advance which youngsters are going to develop the problem and which are not.

Lateral Epicondylitis (Tennis Elbow)

Lateral epicondylitis in the youth is similar to that in the adult. Symptoms can be started by throwing or by racquet sports. Injudicious weight-lifting may also precipitate the problem. The athlete complains of pain over the lateral aspect of his elbow, occasionally associated with swelling. Examination reveals localized tenderness over the lateral epicondyle. Forced extension of the wrist or gripping will cause pain in the same area. X-rays are usually negative but may show soft tissue swelling or some separation of the lateral epicondylar epiphysis.

Treatment is similar to that for little league elbow. Activity must be restricted until the symptoms have disappeared. It is thought that lateral epicondylitis in the tennis player has causes other than elbow overuse. Therefore, inspection of the equipment being used or professional evaluation of the swing should be done to prevent recurrence. Once symptoms have abated, forearm-strengthening exercises using light weights are recommended.

Kienbock's Disease

Osteochondritis of the lunate bone is a problem that affects adolescents. The athlete gives a history of pain in the wrist that may or may not be associated with an injury. Despite adequate treatment, the pain does not resolve. Examination reveals tenderness in the wrist, most marked over the lunate area. Wrist motion is limited. The pain is worse with active motion. X-rays show increased density of the lunate bone in the early stages. In the late stages, collapse and loss of normal architecture occur.

If symptoms are mild and the disease is in its early stages, immobilization in a gauntlet cast for several months may allow revascularization of the lunate. If there has been loss of the normal architecture of the lunate with or without surrounding arthritic changes, surgery may be necessary.

LOWER EXTREMITY PROBLEMS

Slipped Capital Femoral Epiphysis

A slipped epiphysis can be a problem in the athlete from age 9 to the end of growth. It is more common in boys than girls. About one-third of those injured will develop the problem bilaterally. The athlete complains of pain in the hip. Occasionally, the initial complaint may be pain in the knee. A limp develops. Examination reveals an antalgic gait. The youngster is usually overweight, with slow sexual development. In more severe "slips," the athlete's trunk will lean toward the slipped side as weight is put on that limb. Range of motion reveals limitation of internal rotation and abduction of the hip. X-rays of both hips should be taken, since there is a high incidence of bilateral problems. Often the changes in an early slip are subtle but are usually readily seen on the frog-leg view.

Treatment should be in the hands of a specialist. Usually some type of reduction will need to be done by pinning of the epiphysis until growth ceases. In very severe slips, surgery is difficult.

Legg-Perthes' Disease

Osteochondrosis of the femoral epiphysis usually affects boys aged 4–10. It is bilateral in about 15%. The young athlete complains of pain in the hip. There may have been several episodes with complete clearance of symptoms in the interim. The episodes become more frequent and disuse atrophy of the thigh muscles develops. Referred knee pain may be the presenting symptom. Examination reveals loss of thigh musculature and limited abduction and internal rotation. An antalgic gait is usually pronounced. X-rays confirm the diagnosis of the avascular necrosis. Depending on the symptomatology, x-rays may show either the early phase of necrosis, revascularization or bone healing. Femoral epiphysis must go through all these phases before the problem is resolved. Even then, there may be residual deformity.

The principal treatment is to prevent the diseased femoral head from bearing weight. A variety of treatments have been tried, including bed rest, bracing with mobilization and surgery. Because of the judgment involved in treating this problem, it is best handled by a specialist.

Osgood-Schlatter Disease

Pain at the insertion of the patellar tendon on the tibia occurring between the ages of 10–15 is called Osgood-Schlatter disease. The child athlete, usually male, complains of pain and swelling at the tibial tubercle. Often, a direct blow caused the initial problem. The pain is made worse by falling or running. Examination reveals a prominent area over the proximal tibia with localized tenderness. There may be tenderness at the proximal end of the patellar tendon, a symptom of a different entity called "jumper's knee." When the knee is extended against resistance, pain is produced. X-rays occasionally show fragmentation of the tibial tubercle (Fig 8–2). Swelling of the soft tissue is frequently seen.

Initially, the knee should be rested by restricting activities or by splinting until the symptoms have abated. Gradual resumption of activity is allowed. The area should be padded to prevent direct trauma. In some cases the pain is so severe that immobilization in a plaster splint or cast or even enforced bed

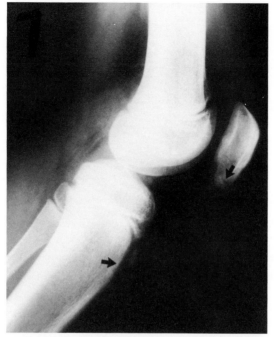

Fig 8–2. — Osgood-Schlatter disease. X-rays often show elevation or fragmentation of the tibial tubercle. Jumper's knee is a painful condition caused by inflammation of the inferior pole of the patella at its junction with the patellar tendon.

rest may be necessary to relieve it. The disease is self-limiting. Usually by the age of 13 in girls and 15 in boys, the problem has spontaneously resolved.

Osteochondritis Dissecans

Avascular necrosis of a portion of the medial femoral condyle is termed osteochondritis dissecans. It can occur in the capitellum, the femoral head and the talus. The most common area is the medial femoral condyle (Fig 8–3). It is more common in boys than in girls, usually young adults. In the early stages the disease is usually not symptomatic; but, as the loose fragment goes through the revascularization phase, intermittent pain associated with some swelling occurs. Examination

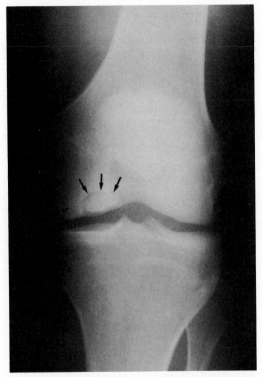

Fig 8–3.—A defect in the medial femoral condyle, indicating osteochondritis dissecans.

reveals mild swelling, probably disuse atrophy of the quadriceps muscles, but normal motion. Tunnel-view x-rays show an isolated fragment of subchondral bone surrounded by a radiolucent line which is often not visible on routine x-rays.

If the defect is not on a weight-bearing surface and not too large, restriction of activity may be all that is necessary. If not, surgery may be necessary.

Chondromalacia of the Patella

Roughness of the articular cartilage underneath the patella is termed chondromalacia. There are several causes, but symptoms are similar. The athlete complains of pain surrounding the kneecap that is usually made worse by going upstairs and much worse by going downstairs. There is often a feeling of fullness or swelling within the knee. Patients whose malacia eventually proves to be secondary to patellar malalignment problems may have additional complaints, such as a vague pain in the knee or a feeling that the knee is slipping or catching.

Examination may be completely normal. However, there may be a mild effusion. There is often subpatellar crepitus, either audible or palpable. Apley's test, performed by displacing the patella distally with the knee extended and having the patient contract his quadriceps, gives a painful, positive result. The relationship of a line from the anterior superior spine of the ilium through the center of the patella to web space between the first and second toes should be observed to determine the relationship of the attachment of the patella tendon. This should not be more than 8–10 degrees. The distance of the inferior pole of the patella from the tibial tubercle should not be much greater than a length equal to that of the length of the patella. X-rays of the knee are usually normal. They may demonstrate patella alta or high-riding patella. Measurement may also indicate an abnormal Q angle (see p. 124), indicating a lateral insertion of the patellar tendon.

There are three possible causes for chondromalacia: trauma, patellar malalignment, and idiopathy. Treatment of all 3 is similar. Initially, the knee must be immobilized for a short period of time until the pain subsides. In early stages there is some indication that aspirin, taken in small doses for a long period of time, will help to smooth the roughened articular cartilage. Static quadriceps exercises followed by weight-lifting with the knee extended are recommended. If this treatment fails, surgery may be indicated.

Shin Splints

Shin splints are more common in youngsters than in adults and usually occur in the early part of the season in running sports. The youth complains of pain over the anterior aspect of his tibia or along the medial flare of the tibia. Any type of strenuous activity causes discomfort. Examination reveals tenderness along the crest of the tibia or along the border of the tibia medially. In more severe cases there will be soft tissue swelling. X-rays are unremarkable.

Rest should be prescribed. Strengthening exercises of the anterior tibial muscles are prescribed when the pain subsides. The athlete should be advised to do warm-up exercises before participating in a sport. After participation, an equal amount of time should be spent in cooling down to help prevent recurrence. In athletes involved in long-distance running, the posterior calf muscles become overdeveloped and shortened, causing a muscle imbalance problem and contributing to shin splints. Be sure that the Achilles tendon group is not tight. If so, stretching of the Achilles tendon will be necessary, in addition to strengthening the anterior muscles.

Achilles Tendinitis

The tendon of the gastro-soleus muscle may become inflamed in children. It is generally caused by overuse, particularly in long-distance running. As running progresses, the gastro-soleus muscle tightens, creating stress on the tendon insertion point on the os calcis. The athlete complains of pain in the area of the insertion, which becomes worse as activity progresses. The tendon may remain sore for several hours to several days following cessation of activity. Examination often reveals tenderness in the area of the insertion of the Achilles tendon. There may be crepitus indicating fluid within the tendon sheath. The tendon sheath itself may be thickened. There is limited dorsiflexion of the foot due to the tight gastro-soleus muscle group.

The tendon must be rested, either by completely restricting activities or by placing the foot and ankle in a cast. When the symptoms have subsided, activity can gradually be resumed. It may be advisable to place a small elevation in the heel of the shoe for several weeks to several months to protect the tendon. Exercises should strengthen the anterior muscles of the leg and stretch the gastro-soleus group. There is no place for the use of anti-inflammatory agents or any injectable drugs in the treatment of children or adolescents.

Sever's Disease

Young athletes who complain of pain just distal to the insertion of the Achilles tendon may have an inflammation of the

apophysis of the os calcis. The athlete complains of pain behind the heel and may have a limp. Examination reveals
tenderness and occasional swelling of the posterior aspect of
the heel. X-rays may show nothing, but they may indicate
increased sclerosis or fragmentation of the apophysis of the
os calcis.

This is a self-limiting problem that may cause symptoms for
a year or more. Padding the heel and slightly elevating it may
make it possible for the athlete to continue in sports.

BACK PROBLEMS

One of the most important things to remember in treating
children's back problems is that youngsters can have herniated nucleus pulposis just like adults. The symptoms will be the
same, and the physical findings are similar. The youthful athlete can sustain back strains similar to the adult, and the treatment is also similar.

The most common children's back problem is spondylolysis, followed by spondylolisthesis (Fig 8–4). Spondylolysis is
the failure of the posterior elements of the spine to develop. It
is most common in the 5th lumbar vertebra and slightly less
frequent in the 4th. If there is a bilateral pars interarticularis
defect or a complete spondylolysis, the upper vertebra can
slip on the lower one, producing spondylolisthesis. Usually
spondylolysis will not be symptomatic, but once slippage has
occurred the back frequently becomes symptomatic. The athlete complains of a low-grade backache, which is made worse
by activity. Pain subsides when the patient lies down.

Examination, including a neurological exam, is frequently
normal. If the physician palpates the spinous process of the
lumbar vertebra carefully, a stepoff may be felt. X-rays will
demonstrate the pars articularis defects on the oblique views.
Any slippage can best be seen on the lateral views. A first-degree slip involves displacement of less than one third of the
width of the vertebra. A slip in the middle third is diagnosed
second degree; third degree if it is beyond that.

If there is a pars articularis defect, but no slippage, or if
there is a first-degree slippage, treatment should include rest
until the pain subsides. Following this, low-back exercises

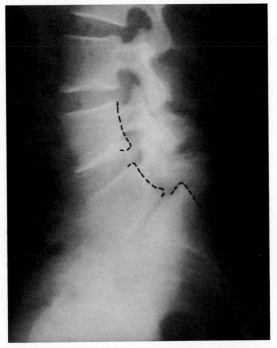

Fig 8-4.—Back pain can be caused by slipping of the 5th lumbar vertebra on the 1st sacral vertebra. X-ray shows a first-degree spondylolisthesis.

should be prescribed. Four to six weeks following clearance of the pain, athletic activities can be resumed. If the problem recurs, or if there is more than a first-degree slip, consultation should be obtained from an orthopedic surgeon before allowing the youth to participate further.

EXERCISE PROGRAMS

In an attempt to increase the strength and/or ability of a prospective young athlete, exercise programs are advised by well-meaning coaches or overenthusiastic parents. It is well for the coach or parent to remember when considering exercise for youngsters that the child is still growing and that the growth centers of the bones are subject to injury from excessive activity or stress. It is not within the scope of this book to set down a specific exercise regimen for each major muscle group. The aim of any program should be to increase endurance, increase strength and maintain flexibility. Amount of weight, the number of repetitions, and the length of the workout should start at a low level and progress gradually to a level that does not produce fatigue. It is probably wise not to allow the youth to lift more than 80% of his weight at any one time or more than 25% of his weight with any one extremity.

A starting point for the amount of weight to be lifted can be ascertained by having the athlete lift what might be considered a minimal weight 8 times. If this can be done without undue fatigue, the same weight should be lifted 15 times. If this can still be done easily, there is not enough weight. If at any point between 8 and 15 fatigue occurs, that is the level at which the athlete should start and the repetitions should be increased gradually to 15. At that level, more weight is added and the repetitions reduced to 8. This cycle is repeated to maximum weight for the child's size. For a 100-lb youngster, 80 lb in a dead lift should be the maximum; 25 lb should be the maximum for an arm or a leg. These general principles should be followed until the athlete has reached skeletal maturity, around 15 in girls and 16 or 17 in boys.

SUGGESTED READING

1. Competitive Athletics for Children of Elementary School Age Joint Committee Statement American Academy of Pediatrics. Pediatrics 42:703, 1968.
2. Shaffer, T. E.: The Adolescent Athlete, Pediatr. Clin. N. Amer. 20: 837, 1973.
3. Tachdjian, M. D.: *Pediatric Orthopedics* (Philadelphia: W. B. Saunders, 1972).
4. Wilmore, J. H.: Adolescence Training to Fit the Sport, Phys. Sports Med. 2:30, 1974.

9 / Nutrition and the Athlete

Few areas in sports medicine are fraught with more myths than those involving nutrition and the athlete. In this chapter we will attempt to explode some of these myths and present a scientifically sound approach to this important aspect of athletics.

BASIC METABOLISM

It is beyond our scope to present an in-depth review of metabolism. However, some fundamentals are necessary if the reader is to have a working knowledge of nutrition.

Protein

The basic components of proteins are the amino acids, which differ from carbohydrates and fatty acids in that they contain nitrogen as well as carbon, oxygen and hydrogen. There are at least 25 different kinds of amino acids, and the body uses about 20 of these to synthesize protein.

The so-called essential amino acids are those that cannot be made from other nutrients (or from other amino acids). Every medical student remembers them from the age-old mnemonic, *Phil V Matt:*

P henylalanine
H istidine
I soleucine
L eucine

V aline

M ethionine
A rginine
T ryptophan
T hreonine

A complete protein, such as that from the muscles of fish, animals and poultry, resembles the amino acid structure of our body's protein. Egg whites have about the best essential amino acid ratio of the common protein-rich foods. One is not limited to these sources of protein, however, for vegetarians can get adequate protein from beans, corn, uncreamed cottage cheese and wheat. Vegetarians should be sure to eat legumes in addition to cereals, for the amino acid lacking in cereal is usually supplied by the legumes.

The athlete often eats protein in excess, erroneously thinking that he is building muscle. Actually, the liver merely strips away the amino group (NH_2) of the excess protein, in a process called deamination, and discards the residua either through fat storage or through the energy cycle. The fate of the residua depends on the structure of the amino acid. Alanine, for example, is called a glucogenic amino acid because, when stripped of its amino group, it becomes part of the glucose metabolic pathway. Minus the amino group, it resembles the glucose unit. A ketogenic amino acid, such as leucine, can form ketone bodies or fat by the active acetate pathway.

The "specific dynamic action" of protein refers to the fact that not all the calories from protein metabolism are available for high-energy adenosine triphosphate (ATP) production. A certain percentage is lost as heat, probably when the carbon-amino bonds are broken. So, on a warm day, it is better for the athlete to eat carbohydrate or fat than protein, since the metabolism of protein releases more heat.

In addition to the foods already mentioned, other good sources of protein include milk and bread (especially bread that is made from high-gluten flour).

Carbohydrates

Basically, carbohydrates are a series of connected carbon atoms which form a simple sugar or a monosaccharide. The three monosaccharides are glucose, fructose and galactose. Dextrose is merely another name for D-glucose.

A disaccharide is produced by combining two simple sugars. There are three different disaccharides:
1. Sucrose table sugar = glucose + fructose
2. Lactose milk sugar = glucose + galactose
3. Maltose = glucose + glucose.

Polysaccharides (starches) are made by joining multiple simple sugars. In the body's energy cycle, glucose is broken down into pyruvic acid and then to active acetate, which has a pivotal role in the process of energy production. If active acetate progresses through the citric acid cycle, the end result is carbon dioxide, water and energy. This process requires oxygen. One unit of the 6-carbon glucose, when processed in this fashion, yields 38 units of high-energy ATP, which in turn can be used to power the essential body processes such as transportation of necessary substances across cell membranes, formation of hormones and various secretions, and the construction of new cells.

Protein, fat and alcohol can also be broken down into active acetate. In addition to the citric acid cycle, active acetate can also be channeled into the production of fatty acids, triglycerides, cholesterol and ketone bodies. Thus, an excess of calories from protein could be metabolized to active acetate and eventually to cholesterol and fat, refuting the theory that a protein diet makes you slim. The various pathways are summarized diagrammatically as follows:

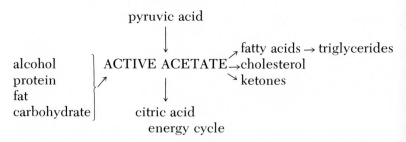

The sedentary obese person uses the fat production (energy-storing) pathway rather than the energy-releasing citric acid cycle.

Fats

Fat is mainly composed of the fatty acid, which is a string of carbon atoms with hydroxyl (OH) groups on the end. If carbon atoms have as many hydrogen atoms attached to them as they can accommodate, they are considered saturated fats. If one or more of the carbon atoms in the chain has an "empty seat," so to speak, it is considered to be an unsaturated fatty acid. If only one of the carbon atoms lacks a hydrogen atom, the fatty acid is considered monounsaturated. If two or more carbon atoms lack a hydrogen atom, the fatty acid is polyunsaturated and cannot be synthesized in humans.

As noted in Chapter 2, the well-trained athlete can rely more on fats for energy needs than on carbohydrates. This is advantageous since fat supplies are more plentiful. The only disadvantage is that it takes more oxygen to get energy from fats than from carbohydrates. As previously mentioned, one molecule of glucose yields 38 ATP units. Fat has an even higher yield: 44 ATP units per molecule of fat metabolized.

The fat in our food is largely triglyceride, which is a combination of three fatty acids with glycerol:

Fatty Acids

The fatty acids in triglycerides may be of the saturated or unsaturated type.

The most prevalent monounsaturated fatty acid in human fat is oleic acid, which constitutes 43% of the fatty acids in humans. Linoleic acid is the major polyunsaturated fatty acid, constituting about 14% of human fatty acids, and can be found in chicken, fish, cooking oils, vegetables and cereals. Linoleic acid is an essential fatty acid, since it is not synthesized in the body. The body can convert linoleic acid into other fatty acids.

Fat in the body is constructed from active acetate units, which we have seen can be derived from protein, carbohydrates, alcohol and dietary fats. Fatty acids are broken down into active acetate when coenzyme A (CoA) hooks onto the end of the fatty acid chain and breaks off two carbon fragments at a time:

$$CH_3-\overset{\overset{\displaystyle O}{\|}}{C}\sim S-CoA$$

active acetate
(acetyl coenzyme A)

The active acetate is quite versatile and can be used in the citric acid cycle to synthesize cholesterol and ketones or to reform fatty acids. The glycerol moiety of triglyceride can be metabolized to glucose, with 100 gm of triglyceride fat yielding 12 gm of blood glucose.

Nearly twice as much cholesterol is formed in the liver from active acetate (1,000–2,000 mg/day) than is taken in by diet (600–1,000 mg/day). It is also formed in the cells lining the intestinal tract. Since cholesterol is contained only in animal foods, its production in humans seems to increase with the dietary intake of saturated fat. Cholesterol can be used to form bile salts and bile acids, which play a role in digestion, and which can be excreted in this form through the gastrointestinal tract. It is also important in the synthesis of adrenal corticosteroid hormones.

It may come as a surprise to many that standard portions (3½ oz or 100 gm) of beef, chicken or certain fish may contain identical amounts of cholesterol (roughly 65–70 mg). The difference is that beef contains higher levels of saturated fats.

The traditional pregame steak is not the ideal food for the athlete, for it contains an abundance of fat, which may stay in the stomach up to several hours after ingestion. The athlete who chooses a high-carbohydrate pregame meal is operating on sounder physiologic and nutritional principles.

Anyone who cooks for an amateur or professional athlete should have a good working knowledge of dietary fats and cooking oils. The most desirable cooking oils are those that are highest in polyunsaturated fat (of which the most common is linoleic acid). The cooking oils can then be graded on their percentage of linoleic acid as follows:

Fat or Oil	% Linoleic Acid
Safflower	75
Sunflower	68
Corn	57
Cottonseed	54
Soybean	50
Sesame	43
Rice bran	32
Peanut	31
Olive	15
Lard	14
Cocoa butter	2
Butterfat	2
Coconut ("vegetable oil")	2

Peanut oil and olive oil contain mainly oleic acid, a monounsaturated fatty acid. Monounsaturates, unlike the saturated fatty acids, do not tend to raise the serum cholesterol level. Polyunsaturated fatty acids, on the other hand, may actually lower the serum cholesterol level.

Soft margarine is preferable to butter because it has a much lower level of saturated fat (17 vs 56%) and a much higher content of polyunsaturated fat (38 vs 3%). In purchasing margarine, one should look for the designation "liquid corn oil" and be wary of those which are listed as "partially hydrogenated." Whole milk and cream should be avoided, because they contain over 50% saturated fat. Mayonnaise and most salad dressings should be excluded from the diet as they contain almost entirely fat calories.

Health food stores promote lecithin, a phospholipid structurally resembling triglyceride, but with a phosphate substituted for a fatty acid and a choline component added. Phospholipids are found in all cells and all cells synthesize this substance, although the liver is the probable source of most of it. About 70% of plasma phospholipid is in the form of phosphatidyl choline (or lecithin), while 20% is in the form of sphingomyelin. Phospholipids are important components of myelin nerve sheaths, play a role in blood coagulation and, as components in bile, help to make fat soluble for absorption. They are major components of plasma lipoproteins, particularly the α-lipoprotein type, and may help stabilize the less polar lipids like cholesterol and triglyceride within the lipoprotein molecule. There is little evidence that lecithin plays a role in the prevention or reversal of atherosclerosis, as claimed by the food faddists, although well-controlled studies in this area would certainly be welcomed.

VITAMINS

Few athletes in the United States are deficient in any of the vitamins if they follow an average diet; yet many feel the need to supplement their diets with expensive commercial preparations.

Vitamin A is essential for normal growth. It plays a role in the formation of adrenal gland hormones, in sperm formation, in the maintenance of skin, hair, teeth, gums and body surface lining cells and is necessary for night vision. It is one of the few vitamins that is stored in the body.

Sources include butter, fortified margarine, milk, eggs and liver. Interestingly, fresh carrots may provide the body with less vitamin A than canned ones, since carrots develop more provitamin A (carotene) as they age. The body can produce vitamin A from carotene, a provitamin found in yellow and dark-green leafy vegetables. Daily doses higher than 5,000 international units (IU) can produce anorexia, irritability, abdominal discomfort, disorders of the skin and hair, bony deposits and "pseudo" brain tumor.

Vitamin B₁ (thiamine) plays a role in the conversion of pyruvic acid to active acetate and is also needed to form the ribose sugar in RNA. It is found in whole-grain or enriched breads, cereals, milk, poultry, fish, pork, lean meat, liver and yeast. The daily requirement is 1.5 mg. The need is slightly greater if the diet is high in carbohydrates. One should also keep in mind that cooking tends to destroy some of the vitamin. A deficiency can produce Wernicke's brain syndrome and beriberi.

Vitamin B₂ (riboflavin) plays a role in the cytochrome *c* energy release process. It is found in the same types of foods that supply vitamin B_1. The daily requirement is 1.8 mg. This vitamin is not significantly affected by heat or cooking but is affected by light. A deficiency of the vitamin might be seen in an alcoholic and can produce soreness of the tongue and cracks in the lips and corners of the mouth.

Vitamin B₆ (pyridoxine), like B_1 and B_2, is found in whole-grain cereals, leafy green vegetables and lean meat. It functions in the transfer of amino groups between carbon structures and in the process of decarboxylation. In addition, it is important in the metabolism of tryptophan, in the formation of red blood cells and in the function of the nervous system. The minimum daily requirement is 2.0 mg. The need is greater when the diet is quite high in protein. Pyridoxine is lost when whole-grain wheat is refined.

Vitamin B₁₂ (cobalamin) is an essential substance for the normal function of all body cells. The vitamins cannot be absorbed in the absence of adequate intrinsic factor, which is produced in the normal stomach but lacking in patients with pernicious anemia. Vitamin B_{12} is particularly important in the production of nucleic acids, which harbor the genetic material, and in the formation of red blood cells. Once-deadly pernicious anemia can now be controlled with regular injections of this vitamin. Dietary sources include milk, foods of animal origin, fish, kidney and liver. The daily requirement is 3 μg.

Niacin (nicotinic acid) is present in all body cells, serving in the energy-producing reactions. It is obtained in meat, liver, eggs, poultry and whole-grain or enriched breads and cereals. Peanuts and peanut butter are excellent sources of niacin. White meat of chicken contains 50% more niacin than does the dark meat. It is found in the husks of cereal grains and is thus removed in the milling process. The body can manufacture it from the amino acid tryptophan. The deficiency state of pellagra (dermatitis, diarrhea, dementia) can develop when individuals follow a corn diet, since the protein in corn is low in tryptophan. Minimum daily requirement will vary with body weight and caloric intake but averages around 20 mg per day.

Vitamin C has received considerable publicity in recent years. It is important in the formation of connective tissue (collagen), bones and teeth. It is not stored in the body, nor can man produce it from carbohydrate substrates as can the cow and the dog. Some claim that large doses of the vitamin reduce the frequency or intensity of colds; recent well-controlled studies refute such claims. Others think that it might be advantageous in combating atherosclerosis, although proof for this theory is lacking. Vitamin C is found in fresh, raw fruits and vegetables. Baked or boiled potatoes are another good source. Vitamin C can be destroyed by copper, iron and possibly cigarette smoke. On the other hand, large doses of vitamin C can destroy much of the vitamin B_{12} ingested. Massive doses of the vitamin can cause diarrhea. Since it is excreted as oxalate, it could also contribute to renal stone formation. The abrupt withdrawal of vitamin C supplements can induce a low blood level. The minimum daily requirement is 45 mg.

Vitamin D is essential for strong teeth and bones. It acts on the intestinal lining to increase the absorption of calcium and phosphorus. It can be found in fortified milk, egg yolk, tuna, salmon and cod-liver oil. The minimum daily need is 400 IU.

Vitamin E (tocopherol) is an alcohol that functions as an antioxidant, preventing oxygen from destroying substances (such as fats) through the formation of toxic peroxides. It can be used as a food preservative because it keeps oxygen from causing fats to become rancid. Vitamin E may play a role in the respiratory chain system and may also help to transmit information from DNA within the cell nucleus to the rest of the cell. It helps to form red blood cells, muscles and other tissues. Sources of vitamin E include whole-grain products, margarine, salad oils, shortening, fruits and vegetables. The minimum daily requirement is 15 IU. Deficiencies of the vitamin produce a variety of diseases in animals. For instance, anemia appears only in monkeys and pigs. Sheep and cows develop heart damage. Vitamin E deficiency rarely, if ever, produces disease in man. Exaggerated claims as to the protective effects of this vitamin on the cardiovascular system are not supported by well-controlled studies. There is no evidence that large doses of vitamin E enhance athletic performance.

Vitamin K is needed to maintain prothrombin and other blood-clotting factors. The major source in man comes from bacterial action in the intestine. Due to a lack of reliable information, a minimum daily allowance has not been established.

Folic acid is vital to the formation of nucleic acids (DNA and RNA) and important coenzymes. It plays a role in cell production and a deficiency can lead to anemia (in this case, a deficiency of red blood cell production). The term "folic acid" refers to its presence in "foliage" (such as spinach leaves). Vegetables, fruits, liver, salads and nuts are other sources. The recommended daily allowance is 400 μg for those over age 10; pregnant women should ingest twice that amount.

MINERALS

A host of minerals are important for normal body function. These include calcium, phosphorus, iron, magnesium, sodium, potassium, chlorine, sulfur and the so-called trace minerals—copper, iodine, zinc, chromium, manganese, fluorine, cobalt, aluminum, bromine, molybdenum, nickel, tin, silicon, selenium and vanadium. In this section we will discuss 5 principal minerals.

Iron, an essential part of hemoglobin and of certain enzyme systems in the body, is necessary for the formation of skin, nails and the lining of the intestinal tract. It is found in leafy green vegetables, egg yolks, meat and liver. Beans are a good source of iron, but unfortunately, the iron in beans is not absorbed as well as the iron in meat. Because an acid environment is needed for iron absorption, Vitamin C enhances this process. The body is able to store up to 5 gm of iron, mainly in the liver. The daily requirement for males under age 18 is 18 mg; it decreases to 10 mg after this age. Menstruating women should consume 18 mg or more per day.

Calcium is necessary for bone and tooth formation, for blood coagulation and for the activity of nerve and muscle cells. Most authorities think that calcium plays a key role in the interaction of myocardial actin and myosin filaments. It is found in fish, hard cheese, milk, butter and egg yolks. The daily need is 1.2 gm up to age 18, then 0.8 gm thereafter. A quart of skim milk provides one and one-half times this amount. Persons who drink hard water may take in an additional 200 mg per day from that source.

Phosphorus is also important in bone and tooth formation and plays a role in muscle contraction and nerve function. It is used to form high-energy substances like ATP and CP (creatine phosphate). Milk, meat and fish are good sources of this mineral, as are whole-grain cereals. The daily requirement is 1.2 gm to age 18 and 0.8 gm thereafter.

Iodine, found in seafood and iodized salt, is an important component of thyroid hormones, which play a role in cell metabolism. The minimum daily requirement is 150 μg.

Magnesium, a metallic element present in almost all cells of the body and in mitochondria, plays a role in the activity of enzymes and in oxidative phosphorylation. It is found in whole-grain cereals, milk, fish, seafood (especially shrimp), vegetables, meat, fruit and nuts. Foods high in both magnesium and oxalate, such as spinach, nuts and wheat germ, may not provide as much magnesium as expected since the oxalate may prevent its absorption. When whole-wheat flour is refined to white flour, 85% of the magnesium is lost. Consequently, 100 gm of whole-wheat flour has 113 mg of magnesium, while a similar amount of white flour has only 25 mg. The daily requirement is 400 mg for those under 18 and 350 mg for those over 18. Reduced serum magnesium levels have been observed after marathon races.

MILK PRODUCTS

A few comments about milk products are in order, as these are often a favorite staple of the athlete. Consider what one glass of skim milk provides, compared to the daily requirement of each ingredient:

Content per Glass	*Daily Need*
Protein – 9 gm	50 – 60 gm
Carbohydrate – 12 gm	200 gm
Fat 0– < 1 gm	50 – 60 gm

Calcium – 300 mg	1000 mg
Iron – 0.1 mg	18 mg
Vitamin A – 10 IU	5000 IU
Vitamin B_1 – 0.09 mg	1.5 mg
Vitamin B_2 – 0.44 mg	1.8 mg
Niacin – 0.2 mg	20 mg
Vitamin C – 2.0 mg	45 mg
Calories – 90	3000 (age 15–22)

Yogurt has gained popularity with certain groups in recent years. It is made by adding bacteria to low-fat milk. The bacteria multiply, converting the lactose in milk to lactic acid. Buttermilk is also made by adding a bacteria (Streptococcus *Lactobacillus*) to skim milk and incubating the mixture until the right acidity is reached.

FIBER

A relentless investigation by Dennis Burkitt,[8] showing that high-fiber diets may protect against many of the common degenerative diseases in man, has popularized this diet. Dr. Burkitt proposes that on a low-fiber diet the bowel bacteria such as Bacteroides and bifidobacteria break down bile acids to lithocholic acids (which act on the liver to decrease the conversion of cholesterol to bile acids, thereby raising the cholesterol content in the body) and to apcholic acid and 3-methylcholanthrene. The latter two are considered possible carcinogens. In a high-fiber diet, the predominant bowel bacteria are Streptococci and Lactobacilli, which cause greater excretion of intact bile acids in the feces. Since cholesterol is a component of bile acids, this may help to reduce the body's cholesterol count. Reducing cholesterol could help to lower the risk of cardiovascular disease.

A reduction of possible carcinogens in high-fiber diets could explain the markedly lower risk of colonic carcinoma in countries with high-fiber diets like Nigeria and Uganda compared to countries with low-fiber diets like the United States and Finland.

These theories are intriguing, but they need some additional study for verification.

SUGAR

Table sugar was unknown to the Greeks and Romans and is not mentioned anywhere in the Bible. Not until the fifteenth century did cane sugar arrive in Europe.

The average American consumes over 100 lb of sugar per year. White sugar provides "empty" calories, that is, it lacks nutrients such as vitamins and minerals. Even brown sugar has only traces of nutrients. Molasses, on the other hand, contains iron, calcium and B vitamins.

Sugar lacks fiber. When eaten in excessive amounts it contributes to dental caries, obesity and possibly to diabetes. Refugees coming from Yemen (where sugar is not readily available) to Israel had virtually no diabetes. A long-term follow-up of these people, now living where sugar is prevalent, showed that up to 5% have developed diabetes.

Yudkin claims that sugar plays a causal role in atherosclerosis, but this theory is not generally accepted by cardiac epidemiologists.

One of the misconceptions in sports nutrition is that honey is particularly healthful. Honey is merely a mixture of two simple sugars, glucose and fructose, and so is similar to table sugar except that it consists of two monosaccharides rather than a disaccharide. The only advantage of using honey over table sugar is to the person who lacks the enzyme sucrase, which is needed to break a disaccharide into monosaccharides. So honey, like molasses and syrups, is a refined carbohydrate.

SALT AND WATER

Since sweat is hypotonic, averaging 50 mEq sodium per liter, the ideal fluid replacement for an athlete should be a hypotonic salt solution with added glucose. The glucose should not exceed 2.5 gm/100 ml (or roughly 6 gm per glass of fluid) since higher levels delay gastric emptying. Most of the commercially available electrolyte "ades" exceed this, ranging from 10 gm of carbohydrates per glass in Gatorade to 22.5 gm per glass in Sportade.

Long-distance runners should not drink more than 1 L of

fluid per hour to avoid fluid retention in the stomach. In warm weather, runners should drink fluids that are slightly chilled to help reduce body temperature.

THE PREGAME MEAL

The concept of the pregame steak, which modern coaches have had difficulty getting away from, dates back to Dromeus of ancient Greece. Dromeus reasoned that by eating the meat of muscular animals, man could develop greater muscles. The fact is that muscle mass is increased by vigorous exercise and not by an exaggerated intake of high-protein foods or supplements. In other words, it is muscle *work*, not vitamins, foods, hormones or drugs, that increases muscle mass. Steak is high in fat and, as mentioned earlier, fat tends to slow the emptying time of the stomach.

A normal, well-balanced meal should be eaten 3 hours prior to an athletic event. Dr. Ralph Nelson, consultant in nutrition at the Mayo Clinic, offers the following sample pregame meal:

Food	Amount
Roast beef	2 oz
Mashed potatoes	½ cup
Dinner roll	1
Margarine	2 tsp
Carrots	½ cup
Skim milk	1 cup
Apple juice	½ cup
Canned peaches	½ cup
Cookies	2

Cooper and Fair prefer a high-carbohydrate meal and recommend orange juice, pancakes (with butter and syrup), dry toast, honey, fruit, fruit cup or Jell-O, milk or tea. They state that "the content of the pregame meal is not critical as long as it does not make the athlete sick or uncomfortable, irritate his GI tract or markedly delay the emptying time of his stomach."

Carbohydrate loading can more than double the muscle glycogen content. The loading procedure is relatively simple—

vigorous exercise while on a low-carbohydrate diet for several days, followed by light exercise and a high-carbohydrate regimen just before an athletic event. The advantage of increased "fuel" for exercise must be weighed against the disadvantage of excessive water deposited in the muscle along with the glycogen. Water could give the sensation of muscle heaviness, while the increased glycogen could destroy muscle fibers, with resultant myoglobulinuria. One 40-year-old distance runner suffered chest pain and ECG abnormalities during carbohydrate loading, raising the question of heart muscle destruction. Until the value and safety of carbohydrate loading are clearly established, we would not advise athletes to undergo self-experiments with this technique.

SUMMARY

Few team physicians are knowledgeable about nutrition, probably because most medical school curricula largely ignore this vital topic. In this chapter we have summarized some of the basic concepts of nutrition, making them relevant to the athlete. Excessive protein does not increase muscle development, contrary to popular belief. About 15% of an athlete's caloric intake should come from protein, 35% from fats (with over half being unsaturated), and 50% from carbohydrates. The latter should be emphasized in the pregame meal, but carbohydrate loading is not generally recommended.

Vitamin supplements are unnecessary. While there is no harm in taking a daily vitamin/mineral preparation, megadoses of vitamins may have adverse effects. Studies have not shown that vitamin C prevents colds nor that vitamin E enhances cardiopulmonary performance.

Lifelong sound nutritional habits can and should be developed in adolescence. The football player of today who stuffs himself with protein supplements, fatty meats, french fries, salt and chocolate sundaes may pay the price in middle age when he is obese, hypertensive, hypercholesterolemic, physically inactive and a prime candidate for a heart attack.

SUGGESTED READING
1. Bergström, J., and Hultman, E.: Nutrition for maximal sports performance, J.A.M.A. 221:999, 1972.

2. Burkitt, D. P., Walker, A. R., and Painter, N. S.: Dietary fiber and disease, J.A.M.A. 229:1068, 1974.

3. Cooper, D. L., and Fair, J.: Pregame meal: to eat or not to eat—and what? Phys. Sportsmed. 4:112, 1976.

4. Dykes, M. H., and Meier, P.: Ascorbic acid and the common cold. Evaluation of its efficacy and toxicity, J.A.M.A. 231:1073, 1975.

5. Harper, H. A.: *Review of Physiological Chemistry* (15th ed.; Los Altos, Calif.: Lange Medical Publications, 1975).

6. Huse, D. M., and Nelson, R. A.: Basic, balanced diet meets requirements of athletes, Phys. Sportsmed. 5:52, 1977.

7. Karlowski, T. R., Chalmers, T. C., Frenkel, L. D., et al.: Ascorbic acid for the common cold. A prophylactic and therapeutic trial, J.A.M.A. 231:1038, 1975.

8. Lamb, L. E.: *Metabolics: Putting Your Food Energy to Work* (New York: Harper & Row, 1974).

9. Mirkin, G.: Carbohydrate loading: A dangerous practice, J.A.M.A. 223:1511, 1973.

10. Nelson, R. A.: What should athletes eat? Unmixing folly and facts, Phys. Sportsmed. 3:67, 1975.

11. Olson, R. E.: Vitamin E and its relation to heart disease, Circulation 48:179, 1973.

12. Rose, L. I., Carroll, D. R., Lowe, S. J., et al.: Serum electrolyte changes after marathon running, J. Appl. Physiol. 29:449, 1970.

13. Shephard, R. J., Campbell, R., Pimm, P., et al.: Do athletes need vitamin E? Phys. Sportsmed. 2:57, 1974.

14. Smith, N. J.: Gaining and losing weight in athletics, J.A.M.A. 236:149, 1976.

Index